FOGSI Focus
Adolescent Intervention for Future Reproductive Health

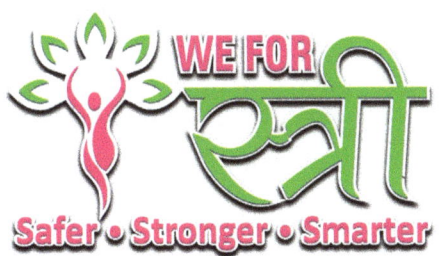

FOGSI Focus
Adolescent Intervention for Future Reproductive Health

Editor-in-Chief
Nandita Palshetkar
MD FCPS FICOG FRCOG (UK)
Professor
Department of Obstetrics and Gynecology
Dr DY Patil Medical College, Hospital and Research Center
Navi Mumbai, Maharashtra, India
Past President, FOGSI, 2019
Scientific Director, Bloom IVF

Editor
Girish Mane
MBBS DGO FICOG
Director
Mane Hospital, Yavatmal, Maharashtra, India
Chairperson
Adolescent Health Committee, FOGSI (2019–2021)
Chairperson
Adolescent Gynecology Committee, AMOGS

Co-Editors

Rohan Palshetkar
MS (Obs and Gyne) FRM
ART Consultant and Endoscopic Surgeon
Associate Professor
Unit Head
Dr DY Patil Medical College, Hospital and Research Center
Navi Mumbai, Maharashtra, India
Joint Treasurer, MAGE; 2nd Joint Secretary, AMOGS
Managing Committee Member, MOGS and MSR

Alok Sharma
MD DHA MICOG
Assistant Professor
Department of Obstetrics and Gynecology
Dr Rajendra Prasad Medical College
Kangra, Himachal Pradesh, India
Founder Secretary Indian Menopause
Society, Shimla Chapter
Founder Secretary Indian Fertility Society, Himachal Pradesh Chapter

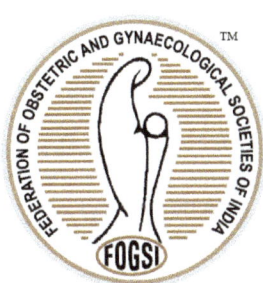

Federation of Obstetric and Gynaecological Societies of India (FOGSI)

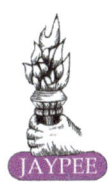

JAYPEE BROTHERS MEDICAL PUBLISHERS
The Health Sciences Publisher
New Delhi | London

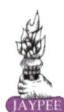 **Jaypee Brothers Medical Publishers (P) Ltd**

Headquarters
Jaypee Brothers Medical Publishers (P) Ltd
EMCA House, 23/23-B
Ansari Road, Daryaganj
New Delhi 110 002, India
Landline: +91-11-23272143, +91-11-23272703
+91-11-23282021, +91-11-23245672
Head Office: 011-43574357
Email: jaypee@jaypeebrothers.com

Corporate Office
Jaypee Brothers Medical Publishers (P) Ltd
4838/24, Ansari Road, Daryaganj
New Delhi 110 002, India
Phone: +91-11-43574357
Fax: +91-11-43574314
Email: jaypee@jaypeebrothers.com

Overseas Office
JP Medical Ltd
83 Victoria Street, London
SW1H 0HW (UK)
Phone: +44 20 3170 8910
Fax: +44 (0)20 3008 6180
Email: info@jpmedpub.com

Website: www.jaypeebrothers.com
Website: www.jaypeedigital.com

© 2021, Jaypee Brothers Medical Publishers

The views and opinions expressed in this book are solely those of the original contributor(s)/author(s) and do not necessarily represent those of editor(s) of the book.

All rights reserved. No part of this publication may be reproduced, stored or transmitted in any form or by any means, electronic, mechanical, photocopying, recording or otherwise, without the prior permission in writing of the publishers.

All brand names and product names used in this book are trade names, service marks, trademarks or registered trademarks of their respective owners. The publisher is not associated with any product or vendor mentioned in this book.

Medical knowledge and practice change constantly. This book is designed to provide accurate, authoritative information about the subject matter in question. However, readers are advised to check the most current information available on procedures included and check information from the manufacturer of each product to be administered, to verify the recommended dose, formula, method and duration of administration, adverse effects and contraindications. It is the responsibility of the practitioner to take all appropriate safety precautions. Neither the publisher nor the author(s)/editor(s) assume any liability for any injury and/or damage to persons or property arising from or related to use of material in this book.

This book is sold on the understanding that the publisher is not engaged in providing professional medical services. If such advice or services are required, the services of a competent medical professional should be sought.

Every effort has been made where necessary to contact holders of copyright to obtain permission to reproduce copyright material. If any have been inadvertently overlooked, the publisher will be pleased to make the necessary arrangements at the first opportunity. The **CD/DVD-ROM** (if any) provided in the sealed envelope with this book is complimentary and free of cost. **Not meant for sale.**

Inquiries for bulk sales may be solicited at: jaypee@jaypeebrothers.com

FOGSI Focus: Adolescent Intervention for Future Reproductive Health

First Edition: 2021

ISBN: 978-93-89776-49-2

Dedicated to

*Dear God, whose eternal blessing and divine presence
helps us to fulfil all our goals*

This book is dedicated to all adolescents.

– **Girish Mane**

Contributors

Aanya Sharma MBBS MD
Resident Doctor (PGY-III)
Department of Obstetrics and Gynecology
Indira Gandhi Medical College
Shimla, Himachal Pradesh, India

Alok Sharma MD DHA MICOG
Assistant Professor
Department of Obstetrics and Gynecology
Dr Rajendra Prasad Medical College
Kangra, Himachal Pradesh, India
Founder Secretary Indian Menopause
Society, Shimla Chapter
Founder Secretary Indian Fertility
Society, Himachal Pradesh Chapter

Bindiya Gupta MD (Obs and Gyne) MAMS FICOG
Associate Professor
Department of Obstetrics and Gynecology
University College of Medical Sciences and Guru Teg
Bahadur Hospital, New Delhi, India

Geetika Gupta Syal MD
Assistant Professor
Department of Obstetrics and Gynecology
Kamla Nehru State Hospital for Mother and Child
Shimla, Himachal Pradesh, India

Girish Mane MBBS DGO FICOG
Director
Mane Hospital
Yavatmal, Maharashtra, India
Chairperson
Adolescent Health Committee, FOGSI (2019–2021)
Chairperson
Adolescent Gynecology Committee, AMOGS

Janki Pandya MS (Obs and Gyne)
Assistant Professor
Department of Obstetrics and Gynecology
AMC-MET Medical College
Sheth Lallubhai Gorthandas General Municipal Hospital
Ahmedabad, Gujarat, India

Jiteeka Thakkar MBBS DGO
Infertility Specialist and Laparoscopic Surgeon
Department of Obstetrics and Gynecology
Kedia Polyclinic
Mumbai, Maharashtra, India

Jitendra Mane MS (Obs and Gyne)
Associate Professor
Department of Obstetrics and Gynecology
Armed Forces Medical College
Pune, Maharashtra, India

Keerti Khetan MBBS MS (Obs and Gyne)
Senior Consultant
Department of Obstetrics and Gynecology
BLK Super Speciality Hospital
New Delhi, India

Manish Machave
MD DNB MNAMS FICOG LLB Dip Endoscopy (Germany) Adv Dip Gyne
Endoscopy (France) Masterclass IIS (Italy)
Gynecologist
Machave Hospital
Pune, Maharashtra, India
Chairperson (Elect)
Ethics and Medicolegal Committee, FOGSI (2020–2022)

MC Patel MBBS DGO FICOG
Gynecologist and Medicolegal Counselor
Niru Maternity and Nursing Home
Ahmedabad, Gujarat, India
Honorary Surgeon
Red Cross Eye Bank, Ahmedabad
Vice President, FOGSI (2018–2019)
Organizing Secretary, AICOG 2017
Organizing Chairperson, MMCON 2018
Honorary Member, Indian Red Cross Society (2019–2021)

Munjal Jayeshkumar Pandya MS (Obs and Gyne)
Assistant Professor
Department of Obstetrics and Gynecology
AMC-MET Medical College
Sheth Lallubhai Gorthandas General Municipal Hospital
Ahmedabad, Gujarat, India

Parag Biniwale MD FICOG FICMCH
Consultant
Department of Obstetrics and Gynecology
Biniwale Multispecialty Clinic
Pune, Maharashtra, India
Secretary
Indian College of Obstetrician and Gynecologist (ICOG)

Priyanka Dilip Kumar
MBBS DNB (OBG) Fellowship in Reproductive Medicine (ICOG)
Consultant
Department of Obstetrics and Gynecology
Fortis Hospital
Bengaluru, Karnataka, India

Rajorhia Anita MBBS MD
Senior Specialist Grade 1 and In-charge
Department of Obstetrics and Gynecology
Sardar Vallabh Bhai Patel Hospital
(Government of NCT of Delhi)
New Delhi, India

Rohan Palshetkar MS (Obs and Gyne) FRM
ART Consultant and Endoscopic Surgeon
Associate Professor
Unit Head
Dr DY Patil Medical College, Hospital and Research Center
Navi Mumbai, Maharashtra, India
Joint Treasurer, MAGE; 2nd Joint Secretary, AMOGS
Managing Committee Member, MOGS and MSR

Roza Olayi MS (Obs and Gyne) MICOG FICOG FICMCH
Director and Consultant and Infertility Specialist
Olyai Hospital
Gwalior, Madhya Pradesh, India
Past Vice President, FOGSI

S Sampathkumari MD DGO FC Dia FICOG FIME
Professor
Department of Obstetrics and Gynecology
Institute of Obstetrics and Gynecology
Madras Medical College
Chennai, Tamil Nadu, India

Santosh Maid MBBS DGO
Director
Dr Maid Hospital
Shirdi, Maharashtra, India

Sheela Mane MBBS MD FICOG FICMCH
Senior Consultant and DNB Teacher
Anugraha Nursing Home
Bengaluru, Karnataka, India

Shilpa Singh MS DNB (Obs and Gyne)
Assistant Professor
Department of Obstetrics and Gynecology
University College of Medical Sciences and Guru Teg
Bahadur Hospital, New Delhi, India

Shyjus Puliyathinkal MBBS MS (Obs and Gyne) (JIPMER) FMAS
DMAS FICOG Certificate in daVinci Robotic Surgical System
Fertility Specialist and Laparoscopic Surgeon
ARMC IVF Fertility Center
Kannur, Kerala, India

Sneha Bhuyar MD
Consultant
Department of Obstetrics and Gynecology
Sukhkarta Hospital
Yavatmal, Maharashtra, India

Suchitra N Pandit
MD DNB FRCOG (UK) FICOG DFP MNAMS B Pharm
Consultant
Department of Obstetrics and Gynecology
Surya Group of Hospitals
Mumbai, Maharashtra, India
Past President, FOGSI

Swati Bhargava MD DNB
Associate Professor
Department of Obstetrics and Gynecology
Government Medical College
Indore, Madhya Pradesh, India

Tripti Sharan MBBS MS (Obs and Gyne)
Senior Consultant
BLK Super Speciality Hospital
New Delhi, India

Vaishali Chavan
MD DGO DNB DFP FICOG Diploma Endoscopy (Germany, France, USA)
Director
Department of Obstetrics and Gynecology
Sahyadri Superspecialty Hospitals and Saanvi Clinic
Pune, Maharashtra, India
Chairperson
Perinatology Committee, FOGSI (2018–2020)

Varsha Lahade MBBS MS FICOG
Gynecologist Class I
Government of Maharashtra, India

President Message

Dear FOGSIANs

The theme of FOGSI this year is "We for Stree". I would like to thank every FOGSIAN who has helped making every woman—Safer Stronger and Smarter. Through various academic and social programs, FOGSI aims to uplift the quality of care that is given to every woman who comes to us.

Adolescent health is an important part of every gynecologist practice. It can be quite challenging and pose a dilemma in our everyday practice. This FOGSI Focus aims at giving you an in-depth update on adolescent health which will help us in our day-to-day practice and also helps us improve adolescent health in the country.

I would like to thank the editors, Girish Mane, Rohan Palshetkar and Alok Sharma for their efforts for bringing out this game wonderful *FOGSI Focus on Adolescent Intervention for Future Reproductive Health*. I would also like to thank all the authors who have contributed towards this FOGSI Focus. I am sure that you will appreciate the effort which has gone into preparing this FOGSI Focus and find them useful in your day-to-day practice.

Wish you all a very happy reading.

Nandita Palshetkar
MD FCPS FICOG FRCOG (UK)
Professor
Department of Obstetrics and Gynecology
Dr DY Patil Medical College, Hospital and Research Center
Navi Mumbai, Maharashtra, India
Past President, FOGSI, 2019
Scientific Director, Bloom IVF

Preface

This particular *FOGSI Focus on Adolescent Intervention for Future Reproductive Health* discusses the details of managing the various physical and mental issues affecting adolescents.

The main aim of this Focus is to ensure that you as gynecologists gets a quick insight and update into adolescent health by reading this focus.

We would like to thank Dr Nandita Palshetkar for giving us this opportunity to be a part of this FOGSI Focus and we hope all of you enjoy reading it as well.

Happy reading!

Thanking you

Girish Mane
Rohan Palshetkar
Alok Sharma

Acknowledgments

Giving thanks is a pleasant job, but it is, nonetheless, difficult when one sincerely tries to put such ideas into words. The following humble words of expression and gratitude cannot really convey the deep feelings of our heart. In any attempt to create and produce a textbook of adolescent gynecology, i.e., *FOGSI Focus on Adolescent Intervention for Future Reproductive Health*, one must be fortunate enough to have the assistance and support of many talented professionals, both within and outside the gynecology department. To begin with, we are indebted to all our authors for their generous contributions to this book; all of them, despite their busy schedules, provided recent, up-to-date, and evidence-based chapters on various aspects of adolescent health for the future perspectives in reproductive health.

We have selected contributors from different parts of India.

It again has been a pleasure to work with the dedicated professionals from M/s Jaypee Brothers Medical Publishers (P) Ltd., New Delhi, India. This publisher has been gracious in offering support without any interference, whatsoever, and the team has also ensured that the quality of work is superb.

We have been deeply indebted to Dr Nandita Palshetkar, Past President FOGSI (2019–2020), for her unconditional support. She has brought her considerable intelligence, energetic work ethic, and creativity to this edition. Her dedication for creating the best textbook possible equalled our efforts to produce an appropriate style for the textbook.

This textbook would not have seen the light of the day without the untiring efforts of Dr Vrishali Mane, who skilfully kept this project on track through an array of potential hurdles.

We acknowledge our respected parents, who have laid the foundation stone of literacy in us and given us the courage to face the challenges of the world by inculcating good attributes in us. We also thank our wives for their tolerance and understanding of the time, we spent away from them during editing this textbook. Their constant encouragement, moral support, and love has been a source of inspiration to us for completing this work. Finally, but certainly not last, we thank our children for their immense patience.

Contents

1. Thieves of Sexual Health, Future Fertility and Reproductive Outcomes in Adolescents 1
   Roza Olayi, Rajorhia Anita

2. Adolescent PCOS: The Hunter for Dolls 7
   S Sampathkumari

3. Primary Amenorrhea 11
   Alok Sharma, Geetika Gupta Syal, Aanya Sharma

4. Congenital Anomalies: Future Fertility! 16
   Shyjus Puliyathinkal

5. Fertility Preservation in Ovarian Tumors in Adolescents 22
   Tripti Sharan, Keerti Khetan

6. Uterine Fibroids in Adolescents 28
   Priyanka Dilip Kumar

7. Endometriosis in Adolescents 31
   Sheela Mane

8. Menstrual Abnormalities in Adolescents 36
   Jitendra Mane, Parag Biniwale

9. Teenage Pregnancies and Abortions: Today's Scenario 42
   Munjal Jayeshkumar Pandya, Janki Pandya

10. Anemia in Adolescents 48
    Shilpa Singh, Bindiya Gupta

11. Sexually Transmitted Infection in Adolescents 53
    Suchitra N Pandit, Swati Bhargava

12. Contraception in Adolescents 60
    Girish Mane, Santosh Maid

13. Sexual Reproductive and Health Rights in Adolescents 64
    Rohan Palshetkar, Jiteeka Thakkar

14. The Protection of Children from Sexual Offences Act, 2012 (POCSO):
    What Every OB-GYN Specialist should Know? 66
    MC Patel, Manish Machave

15. Premarital Sex and Unprotected Sexual Activity in Adolescents 69
    Sneha Bhuyar

16. Adolescent-friendly Health Clinics 74
    Vaishali Chavan, Varsha Lahade

Index 77

CHAPTER 1

Thieves of Sexual Health, Future Fertility and Reproductive Outcomes in Adolescents

Roza Olayi, Rajorhia Anita

■ INTRODUCTION

Adolescence is a challenging period in life of an individual and envisages development of new relationships and behaviors that persist throughout life. As per WHO, the world now has more young than past and adolescents are one-sixth of the world's population and make around 42% of the young population worldwide. The clinicians attending to these adolescents face unique challenge, while dealing with this age group, due to their varied and complex physical, psychological, social, gynecological and sexual health concerns.

The concern for future fertility and sexual health may be paramount in this age group. The clinicians need to be well versed with their concerns and must be trained enough to counsel about these. There are many factors which may have a large impact on future fertility and sexual health of adolescent age group and require timely interventions to prevent future permanent implications of these conditions.

The various factors which may act as stealers or thieves of future fertility and sexual health of adolescents are as follows; some conditions may fall in the categories of more than one class.[1-6,10-12]

- *Genetic*:
  - *Kallmann's syndrome:*
    - Mutations in the follicle-stimulating hormone (*FSH*) beta gene
    - Turner's syndrome (45 XO)
    - Galactosemia
  - Klinefelter's syndrome (47-XXY)
  - *46 XX primary ovarian deficiency:*
    - Down's syndrome
    - Fragile-X permutation
    - 46 XX gonadal dysgenesis
    - Mutation of sex-determining region of Y chromosome (SRY) such as Swyer's syndrome
  - Cystic fibrosis

- *Congenital and acquired anatomical abnormalities*:
  - Congenital absence of uterus and vagina
  - Imperforate hymen
  - Anorectal malformations
  - Transverse vaginal septum
  - Cervical atresia
  - Mullerian dysgenesis (MRKH syndrome)
  - Absolute uterine factors and other Mullerian anomalies
  - Asherman's syndrome
  - Endometriosis
  - Fibroids
  - Genital mutilation
  - Spina bifida or spinal injuries
  - Cerebral palsy
  - Bilateral cryptorchidism
  - Anorchia/Testicular regression
- *Receptor and enzyme defects*:
  - Congenital adrenal hyperplasia (17 alpha-hydroxylase deficiency)
  - Androgen insensitivity syndrome due to defective androgen receptor
  - FSH, luteinizing hormone (LH) inactivating mutations leading to gonadotropin resistance
  - Aromatase deficiency
- *Growth and development problems*:
  - Isolated gonadotropin-releasing hormone (GnRH) deficiency
  - Hypopituitarism
  - Constitutional delay of puberty
  - Congenital central nervous system defects
  - Age-related fecundity decline
- *Metabolic and endocrinological problems*:
  - Polycystic ovary syndrome (PCOS)
  - Obesity
  - Congenital adrenal hyperplasia

- Diabetes mellitus
- Hypothyroidism and hyperthyroidism
- Cushing's syndrome
- Hypogonadotropic hypogonadism
- Transgender
- Pseudohypoparathyroidism
- Hyperprolactinemia
- Autoimmune ovarian insufficiency and premature ovarian failure
- Empty sella and Sheehan's syndrome
- Prader-Willi's syndrome and leptin deficiency

- *Neoplasia/tumors*:
  - Craniopharyngioma
  - Pituitary adenoma
  - Ovarian tumors
  - Testicular tumors
  - Childhood cancer survivors of acute lymphoblastic leukemia, acute myeloid leukemia, non-Hodgkin lymphoma, neuroblastoma, soft tissue, and germ cell tumors

- *Infections*:
  - Mumps
  - Chronic pelvic inflammatory diseases, e.g., chlamydia
  - Sexually transmitted infections (STIs)
  - Vulvovaginitis
  - Genital tuberculosis
  - Malaria
  - HIV/AIDS
  - Human papillomavirus (HPV) infection
  - Postpartum and postabortal sepsis (unsafe abortions)

- *Immunological and rheumatological*:
  - Lupus/mixed connective tissue disease
  - Vasculitis
  - Steroid-dependent nephrotic syndrome
  - Rheumatoid arthritis

- *Other chronic ailments*:
  - End-stage renal disease
  - End-stage liver disease
  - End-stage cardiac disease
  - End-stage lung disease
  - Dermatological conditions—anogenital warts, lichen planus, lichen sclerosis

- *Environmental and social*:
  - Poor socioeconomic status
  - Genital trauma and mutilation
  - Poor perineal hygiene and menstrual hygiene
  - Use of local irritants, e.g., feminine sprays, soaps, perineal wash, etc.
  - Availability of clean toilets in schools and public places
  - Dietary factors—over nutrition and under nutrition
  - Use of tobacco and smoking
  - Excessive caffeine use, alcohol intake and drug abuse
  - Sexual abuse and violence
  - Exercise and extreme sports activities
  - Immunization status, e.g., HPV, etc.
  - Education level, gender bias, family, and partner support
  - Local cultural, religious, political factors
  - Legislation around age of marriage and employment
  - Environmental toxin exposer and endocrine disrupting chemicals (EDCs)
  - Preconception care and interventions
  - Accessibility and availability of adolescent reproductive and sexual health (ARSH) program and fertility preservation facilities

- *Mental and psychological state*:
  - Psychological stress
  - Depression
  - Anxiety
  - High-risk behavior
  - Sexuality
  - Eating disorders
  - Dating violence
  - Poor mental health literacy and attending mental health services

- *Adolescent responsive quality healthcare*:
  - ARSH program and sexual and reproductive health services
  - Poor treatment adherence—role of apps and other web-based technology
  - Fertility preservation services
  - Preconception counseling and care during pregnancy
  - Availability of HIV/AIDS, tuberculosis and STI treatment
  - Mental health services
  - School-based health services
  - Vaccination for measles, rubella, BCG, Hepatitis-B vaccine, diphtheria-tetanus, influenza, HPV, etc.

- *Iatrogenic*:
  - *Gonadotoxic chemotherapy*: Alkylating agents, heavy metals
  - *Gonadotoxic radiotherapy*: Pelvic irradiation
  - Surgical extirpation of uterus and ovaries, Fallopian tubes for various indications
  - Orchidectomy.

ASSESSMENT OF ADOLESCENTS FOR FUTURE FERTILITY

The parents of or chronically-ill adolescents may seek inquiry about scope of their future fertility. A systematic history, examination and investigations may be required for prognostication.[13]

History

A careful history taken in a very empathetic and confidential way is important which includes:
- Detail childhood growth and development
- Age at thelarche
- Age at menarche
- Any history of cyclical pelvic pain or prolonged pain in lower abdomen
- Detailed menstrual history
- Any history of amenorrhea
- Dysmenorrhea or abnormal uterine bleeding
- Past history of alcohol intake
- Any drug intake for prolonged illness
- History of any pelvic or perineal trauma, sexual abuse or violence
- History of smoking or tobacco use or substance abuse
- Sexual history, if relevant and contraceptive use and medical termination of pregnancy done in past
- Any history of irradiation to pelvis in past
- Any history of surgery done in pelvic area
- Dietary history
- History of any psychiatric illness or medication taken for same
- History of excessive hair growth over body or face
- History of galactorrhea, thyroid disease, pituitary or adrenal disease diabetes, tuberculosis, sexually transmitted diseases
- Any history of hot flushes, anxiety, sleep disturbance, night sweats is to be elicited
- Headache or visual field changes
- Any history of bleeding disorder in the adolescent or family
- History of genetic diseases and familial caners in the next of kin
- History of HIV, AIDS, Hepatitis
- Chronic kidney disease.

Examination

A thorough physical examination of adolescent is required which includes looking for:
- Height
- Weight
- Body mass index (BMI)
- Thyromegaly
- Lymphadenopathy
- Tanner staging and breast development
- Systemic examination including respiratory, cardiovascular, neurological system
- Vision and visual field
- Blood pressure
- Signs of virilization/hirsutism
- Striae and pigmentation
- Examination of inguinal canal for any palpable gonads
- Urological and genital tract examination in both male and female adolescent
- Testicular volume by Prader orchidometer
- Evaluation in relevant cases for psychological age as against chronological age.

Investigations

These may be required both for diagnosis of underlying clinical conditions that affect fertility and their follow-up and prognostication of future fertility and reproductive outcomes.
- Hemogram and platelet count
- Erythrocyte sedimentation rate
- Screening for diabetes
- Thyroid function tests
- S prolactin
- FSH, LH, anti-Müllerian hormone (AMH), serum estradiol
- S testosterone, dehydroepiandrosterone sulfate
- Androstenedione, 17-OH progesterone
- Coagulation profile and vonWillebrand disease panel
- Kidney function test
- Liver function test
- Abdominal and pelvic ultrasound
- Magnetic resonance imaging for pituitary and hypothalamus
- Tests for bone age
- Karyotype
- Tumor marker in suspected malignancies, e.g., CA 125, alpha fetoprotein, beta hCG, carcinoembryonic antigen and lactate dehydrogenase, etc.

Counseling

It incorporates involvement of gynecologist, andrologist, geneticist, infertility/IVF specialist, and psychiatrist. Adolescents are made aware about their future fertility concerns along with parents initially and later in separate sessions as per requirement of confidentiality. Fertility awareness is generated in adolescents and their misconceptions and doubts are cleared regarding their reproductive and sexual health. This empowers adolescents to make informed reproductive choices and helps them to optimize their future fertility.[7] A culture appropriate counseling is done to help parents overcome their emotional turmoil first so that they may help the adolescent later on in dealing with their self-esteem and body image issues in spite of their subfertility in certain conditions.

Adolescents are counseled about modifiable risk factors for infertility and are advised to make lifestyle modifications to conserve and preserve their future fertility and reproductive outcomes. They are given nutritional counseling and deficiencies are corrected. Adolescents are empowered to stop smoking, tobacco use, caffeine and alcohol intake in adequate number of counseling sessions. They are advised to optimize their BMI and moderate exercises are encouraged keeping into consideration their underlying clinical disease and exercise tolerance. Effort should be made to minimize their exposure to environmental toxins, EDCs and self-harming practices. The importance of good psychological assistance, support to allay stress and anxiety, and cognitive behavioral therapy, as and when required, cannot be underemphasized to maintain optimism for future fertility. Counseling about availability of fertility preservation options is important and is discussed ahead.[9]

Transgender adolescents pose challenges to counselors as their concern may depend on their parenthood desires, family perceptions about biological child, fertility information specific to them and finances involved in the process.[8]

MANAGEMENT OF SOME COMMON STEALERS OF FUTURE FERTILITY

Reproductive Tract Anomalies

Anomalies of female genital tract may be due to agenesis/hypoplasia, vertical fusion or canalization, and contact abnormalities with urogenital sinus, lateral fusion defects or resorption. Adolescents may present with amenorrhea, pain in lower abdomen or pelvis, unhealthy vaginal discharge or abnormal vaginal bleeding specially with obstructive anomalies. Adolescents into acute abdomen may be diagnosed with obstructive anomalies and need surgical intervention.

Many Mullerian anomalies remain undiagnosed during adolescence. They may present later on in life, when pregnancy is contemplated, with either recurrent pregnancy loss or infertility. Diagnosis of Mullerian agenesis may be a traumatizing experience to the adolescent or her family. Counseling by expert team is important as already mentioned and family should be informed about potential reproductive function due to normal ovarian function, including production of sex steroids and fertility options of assisted reproduction technologies and surrogacy is discussed. Creation of neovagina is delayed till adolescent is mature enough to understand nature of treatment and its timing. Most uterine fusion defects do not require surgical correction until there is specific concern of poor reproductive outcome in form of infertility or recurrent pregnancy loss. Absolute uterine factors may need surrogacy.

Sexually Transmitted Diseases

Adolescent females are more prone to develop sexually transmitted diseases than adult females and males. They may have asymptomatic infection and may not seek health care due to sociocultural barriers. This may have long-term reproductive implications, as may later on lead to pelvic inflammatory disease, which is an important cause of infertility and ectopic gestation. Timely diagnosis and treatment of STI such as *Neisseria gonorrhoeae*, chlamydia, trichomoniasis can prevent this. Young, sexually active adolescents may develop HPV infection. Persistence of high risk subtypes of HPV with oncogenic potential may lead to development of high grade cervical intraepithelial neoplasia and carcinoma cervix, if screening and timely intervention is not done HPV vaccination can prevent this dreadful consequence which may cause subfertility and may be fatal.

Abnormal Uterine Bleeding

Abnormal uterine bleeding due to varied causes, as discussed earlier, may give a hint to underlying pathology which may affect later fertility in adolescents. A careful evaluation needs to be done as per PALM-COEIN classification and cause specific treatment is instituted, as abnormal uterine bleeding may indicate irregular ovulation and dwindling fertility later on in life. Adolescents need correction of associated anemia for general health well-being and better reproductive outcomes later on in life.

Polycystic Ovary Syndrome and Other Conditions Associated with Hyperandrogenemia

Counseling of PCOS patients should be started early in adolescence regarding life style management to avoid development of metabolic syndrome later on in life. Metabolic syndrome can compromise fertility. PCOS itself causes infertility due to associated oligo-ovulation or anovulation. The association of unopposed estrogen exposure to development of endometrial hyperplasia and endometrial cancer later on in life may hamper fertility due to clinical condition itself or due to treatment given for the same, which may need medical or surgical interventions. Overzealous treatment of PCOS by ovarian drilling may itself cause decreased ovarian reserve, ovarian in-sufficiency and premature ovarian failure, so it must be avoided except in specific situations associated with infertility in late adolescence.

Endometriosis

Young adolescents may be diagnosed with this disease when their chronic pelvic pain does not respond to nonsteroidal anti-inflammatory drugs. Endometriosis in adolescents is usually associated with some obstructive Mullerian anomaly. As endometriosis is a progressive disease, patient may later on develop endometriomas and deep infiltrating endometriosis which may cause infertility due to decreased ovarian reserve, distortion of pelvic anatomy and disturbed tubo-ovarian relationship. Goal of therapy in young adolescents is symptomatic relief, suppression of disease progression, and protection of future fertility. Medical management with oral contraceptive pills, progestin therapy or GnRH agonist is preferred and surgery in adolescents is reserved only for patients who do not respond to medical management of chromic pelvic pain. As such, due to inherent progressive nature of disease, she may need multiple surgeries later on in life, may be as a part of infertility management. Patient can be put on continuous hormonal suppression till she is desirous of and contemplates pregnancy. Surgical treatment involves fulguration or complete excision of clear white vesicular and red lesions. Cystectomy, if needed, should involve complete cyst removal except near hilum to preserve ovarian reserve. Levonorgestrel-releasing intrauterine device (LNG-IUD) may be inserted at the time of laparoscopy to prevent recurrence of disease or patient may be given medical treatment as discussed before or etonogestrel subdermal implant may be given.[14]

Ovarian Cysts and their Torsion

Adolescents may present with simple or complex ovarian cysts. Conservative approach is desirable in form of simple observation or organ sparing surgery to protect their future fertility. Simple cysts less than 6 cm may be observed with or without giving combined oral contraceptive pills for around 3 months, to prevent recurrence. Cysts more than 10 cm will not regress usually and need laparoscopic intervention. Ovarian cysts may undergo torsion and may need conservative surgery in form of untwisting of ovarian pedicle and simple observation. Cystectomy at same sitting is avoided as it may lead to more traumas of friable ovarian tissues. The untwisted ovary usually regains its functions and looks normal on follow-up.[15]

Hemorrhagic cysts need observation and surgical treatment only in exceptional cases to protect fertility.

Adolescents with Cancer

Oncofertility is a developing science. Survivors of childhood cancers and newly diagnosed adolescents with hematological or genital malignancy will need comprehensive reproductive evaluation and follow-up regarding ensuing gonadal insufficiency, sexual dysfunction, and infertility. The disease itself or its management may cause disturbances in attainment of puberty which may be precocious or may get delayed.

As there is finite number of follicles in ovary, there may be age-related decline in fertility. Moreover, adolescents receiving alkylating agents such as cyclophosphamide and procarbazine or heavy metals as chemotherapeutic agents, have detrimental effect on their ovarian reserve in dose dependent and cumulative way. Prepubertal or pubertal gonadal irradiation may be a risk factor for hypogonadism. Older adolescents, due to their less number of oocyte stores, may develop acute ovarian failure (within 5 years of cancer treatment) or premature menopause or primary ovarian insufficiency. This causes sexual dysfunction due to vulvovaginal cicatrization or narrowing, dysfunction of ovary in form of dwindling hormonal function, and less lubrication and dryness caused by vestibular gland dysfunction.

It is prudent to discuss future fertility concerns at the start of cancer treatment to avoid any repentance later on. All "fertility preservation options" such as oocyte cryopreservation, ovarian cortex cryopreservation are discussed with adolescent and family. Option of embryo cryopreservation is offered if the adolescent has a partner. Some experimental studies are going on in vitro maturation of immature oocytes retrieved without any ovarian stimulation.

Ovarian transposition or oophoropexy before pelvic irradiation may be offered but future reproductive outcome is not ensured as uterus is not protected and may have irreversible endometrial and blood supply damage.

Studies are going on about use of GnRH agonist use during chemotherapy to quieten the ovary, as it will suppress ovarian function and decrease blood supply, minimizing the exposure of ovary to chemotherapeutic agents but results are not favoring it as standalone option. Menstrual lightening may be tried with combined hormonal contraceptives, LNG-IUD or depot medroxyprogesterone acetate injections. This will correct anemia of patient as well and provide contraception during cancer treatment as added advantage.

Male adolescents are offered sperm cryopreservation.

The follow-up assessment for fertility potential should continue closely during and after cancer treatment. The ethical and social issues of fertility cryopreservation must be discussed with parents and adolescents, as some adolescents later on in life may not be well enough to provide optimum parenting due to health issues and some may unfortunately not survive till embarking on conception.[16-18]

CONCLUSION

Most adolescents expect to have their biological children in future if properly counseled and given an option. The prognosis of fertility potential in future will depend upon underlying pathophysiology of their disease and effect of its treatment involved. The thieves and stealers of reproductive future of adolescents can only be conquered by timely diagnosis and management of the disease and therapy optimization. Fertility preservation option should be offered to adolescents diagnosed with cancer. Expert quality counseling regarding perception and priorities of adolescents about decision making for future fertility is the corner stone of treatment.

REFERENCES

1. Rossi BV, Abusief M, Missmer SA. Modifiable risk factors and infertility: what are the connections? Am J Lifestyle Med. 2016;10(4):220-31.
2. Sanfilippo JS, Lara-Torre E. Adolescent gynecology. Obstet Gynecol. 2009;113(4):935-47.
3. Hertweck P, Yoost J. Common problems in pediatric and adolescent gynecology. Expert Review Obstet Gyne. 2010;5(3):311-28.
4. DeSapri KAT, Lucidi RS. What are the differential diagnoses for Amenorrhea? [online] Available from: https://www.medscape.com/answers/252928-35725/what-are-the-differential-diagnoses-for-amenorrhea. [Last accessed November, 2019].
5. Hallgarten A. Revolutionising reproduction: the future of fertility treatment. [online] Available from: https//www.bionews.org.uk/page-142170. [Last accessed November, 2019].
6. Fertility factor (demography). [online] Available from: https://en.wikipedia.org/wiki/Fertility_factor_(demography). [Last accessed November, 2019].
7. Kudesia R, Talib HJ. Fertility counseling for adolescents. Pediatric Annals. 2019;48(2):e86-91.
8. Chen D, Kyweluk MA, Sajwani A, Gordon EJ, Johnson EK, Finlayson CA. Factors affecting fertility decision-making among transgender adolescents and young adults. LGBT Health. 2019;6(3):107-15.
9. World Health Organization. Global Accelerated Action for the Health of Adolescents (AA-HA!): guidance to support country implementation coming of age adolescent health. Maternal, newborn, child & adolescent health. [online] Available from: https://www.who.int/maternal_child_adolescent/topics/adolescence/framework-accelerated-action/en/. [Last accessed November, 2019].
10. Centers for Disease Control and Prevention. Common reproductive health concerns for women reproductive health. MedlinePlus.
11. Mmari K, Blum RW. Risk and protective factors that affect adolescent reproductive health in developing countries: a structured literature review. Glob Public Health. 2009; 4(4):350-66.
12. Adolescent sexual reproductive health. Child & adolescent health & development. World Health Organization website.
13. Gillam ML. Gynecologic problems of adolescence and puberty. [online] Available from: https://www.glowm.com/section_view/heading/Gynecologic%20Problems%20of%20Adolescence%20and%20Puberty/item/13. [Last accessed November, 2019].
14. ACOG committee opinion. Dysmenorrhea and endometriosis in the adolescent. [online] Available from: https://www.acog.org/Clinical-Guidance-and-Publications/Committee-Opinions/Committee-on-Adolescent-Health-Care/Dysmenorrhea-and-Endometriosis-in-the-Adolescent?IsMobileSet=false. [Last accessed November, 2019].
15. Murat OZ, Yakut HI, Ozgu BS, Ozgu E, Korkmaz E, Gungor T. Adolescent gynaecology: satisfying the needs for special patients. OA Women's Health. 2014;2(1):1.
16. Levine JM. Preserving fertility in children and adolescents with cancer. Children (Basel). 2014;1(2):166-85.
17. Peddie VL, Porter MA, Barbour R, Culligan D, MacDonald G, King D. Factors affecting decision making about fertility preservation after cancer diagnosis: a qualitative study. BJOG. 2012;119(9):1049-57.
18. Gylynthia ET, Hoefgen Holly. Gynecologic issues in the pediatric and adolescent patient with cancer. Curr Treat Options Peds (2016) 2:196-208. Pediatric Gynecology (L Breechand K Stambough, Section Editors). Published online: 19 July 2016. DOI 10.1.

CHAPTER 2

Adolescent PCOS: The Hunter for Dolls

S Sampathkumari

INTRODUCTION

Polycystic ovary syndrome (PCOS) affects women from menarche to menopause causing multiple problems. This condition affects their petite stature leading to obesity, hirsutism, acanthosis, thereby disfiguring their doll like appearance. PCOS thus hunts women throughout their life resulting in infertility, stress over appearance, anxiety. It is important for us to intervene and hunt the hunter before it can cause permanent damage to the future of these women. Adolescence is the apt time to attend to this problem without further aggravating the issue in her other stages of life.

Adolescence is the period from onset of prepubertal changes, attaining puberty, and adapting to pubertal changes. Polycystic ovary in adolescence presents with complaints of hirsutism, menstrual irregularity and/or obesity. This is a common condition and leading cause of infertility in later days.

ETIOPATHOGENESIS

Polycystic ovary syndrome involves ovulatory dysfunction and increased androgen synthesis. Defects in ovarian steroidogenesis form the pathophysiology of PCOS (**Fig. 1**). It has genetic basis too and is inherited as autosomal dominant with variable penetrance.[1] Anovulation leads to irregular menstrual cycles with cycle length varying from 19 to 90 days. Inappropriate gonadotropin secretion, with changes in follicle stimulating hormone (FSH) and luteinizing hormone (LH), lead on to ovulatory dysfunction. This forms a cycle due to loss of negative feedback. Also, impaired ovarian steroidogenesis leads to increased androgen production from ovarian stroma and theca call hyperplasia. Occurrence of insulin resistance leads to hyperinsulinemia. Decreased sex hormone binding globulin by action of liver in turn causes increasing of free androgen levels. Insulin resistance also alters the lipid and glucose metabolism.

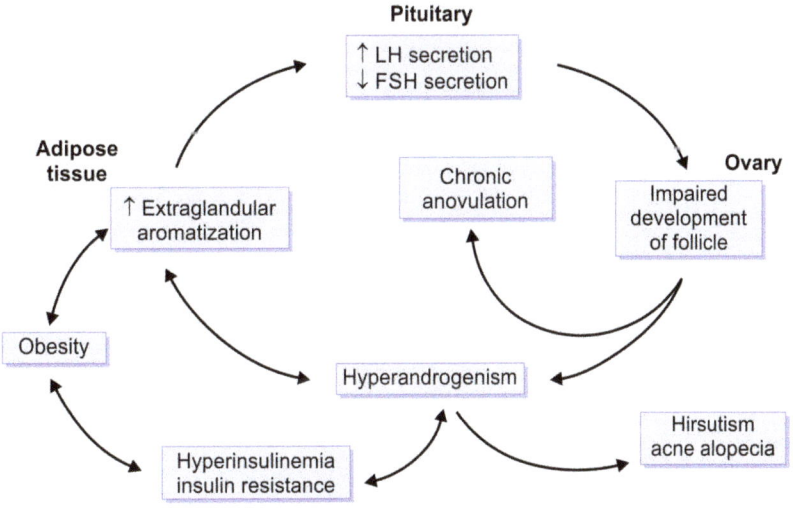

Fig. 1: Pathophysiology of PCOS.
(FSH: follicle stimulating hormone; LH: luteinizing hormone; PCOS: polycystic ovary syndrome)

CLINICAL FEATURES
- Irregular menstrual cycles
- Obesity
- Insulin resistance
- Hirsutism
- Acne

Adolescents tend to have anovulatory cycles initially due to immaturity of hypothalamo pituitary axis. However, in the presence of hyperandrogenism, persistent anovulation for >2 years, the likelihood of having PCOS is >80%.[2] In the absence of any endocrine disorder, persistent anovulatory cycles >1 year presenting as irregular menstrual cycles is 50% likely due to PCOS in adolescent.

Sexual hair growth is graded by Ferriman-Gallwey scoring system **(Fig. 2)**. Scores 8-15 indicate mild hirsutism and 16-24 indicate moderate hirsutism.[3] This scoring system assesses hair growth in 9 areas and scores 0 (no hair) to 4 (abundant virile hair) in each area. This is difficult for an adolescent because they have not attained sexual maturity and sexual hair growth is in process of development.

Acne is a common manifestation of puberty. This is mostly comedonal acne. Moderate to severe inflammatory acne is not a common manifestation and it indicates PCOS. This kind of persistent acne that is unresponsive to topical treatments need to be evaluated for hyperandrogenism before starting on oral contraceptive pills (OCPs), because OCPs can mask features of PCOS. Comedonal acne refers to blackheads or whiteheads >1 mm diameter. Inflammatory acne present as pustules, papules <5 mm, nodules >5 mm, with scarring. Examination of face, chest, back, and shoulders for acne is advised.

Normal upper limits for total testosterone are 55 ng/mL and free testosterone is 9 pg/mL. Free testosterone is a more reliable indicator of hyperandrogenism than total hormone. However, elevated levels in asymptomatic girls have no significance. Only when this increased levels present with persistent anovulation, it is diagnostic of PCOS.

Ultrasonographic picture of ≥12 small antral follicles (2-9 mm diameter) per ovary with ovarian volume >10 mL per ovary characterizes appearance of polycystic ovaries. There is ovarian enlargement, thecal hyperplasia, capsular thickening, and luteinization. However, it is difficult to count antral follicle count with abdominal scan in adolescents and also 50-75% adolescents generally meet the adult criteria as

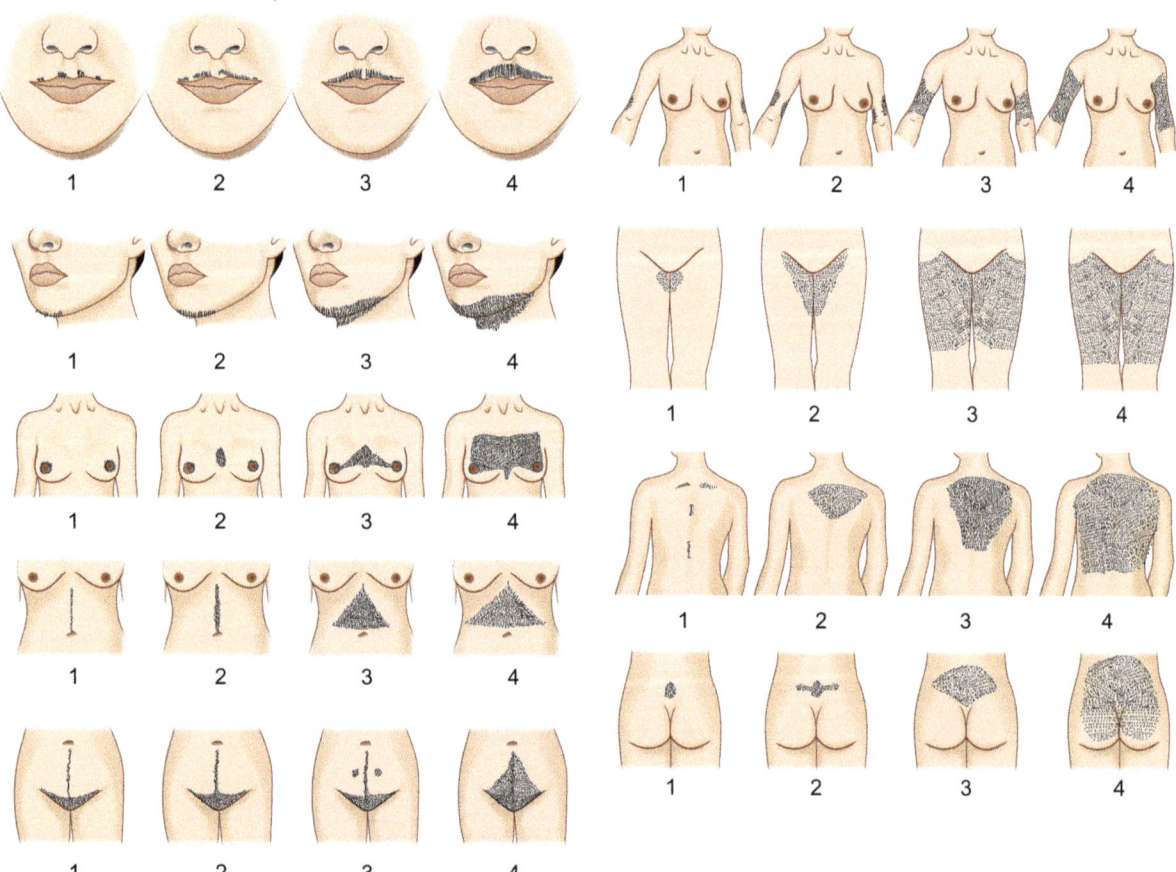

Fig. 2: Ferriman–Gallwey score.

normal variant.[4] So, mean ovarian volume >12 cc or single ovary >15 cc is considered enlarged for adolescent.[5]

Insulin resistance can be present in both obese and nonobese PCOS. Obesity is present in about 50% PCOS patients.[6] Insulin resistance results in increased abdominal fat deposits irrespective of body mass index status. It can manifest as acanthosis nigricans. But PCOS can present without insulin resistance or obesity also.

COMPLICATIONS

- Infertility
- Metabolic syndrome
- Type 2 diabetes mellitus
- Cardiovascular disease risk
- Endometrial cancer

Metabolic syndrome which is a group of conditions ranging from central obesity, glucose abnormality, hypertension, dyslipidemia occurs in 25% PCOS individuals.[5] This leads to type 2 diabetes mellitus, cardiovascular risk, and sleep apnea disturbances as they progress to adulthood.

DIAGNOSIS

The Rotterdam criteria for PCOS in adult are unexplained hyperandrogenism, anovulation, and ultrasound picture of polycystic ovaries. However, using these criteria to diagnose PCOS in adolescent is difficult as anovulation and acne are common in adolescents. So, the Pediatric Endocrine Society has come up with following criteria for diagnosing PCOS in adolescent.

Combination of unexplained abnormal uterine bleeding (AUB) and hyperandrogenism[7] can lead to persistent AUB for 1 or 2 years. Hyperandrogenism can be diagnosed clinically as moderate to severe hirsutism, moderate to severe acne vulgaris refractory to treatment, androgenic alopecia, and laboratory values of serum testosterone elevated above normal limits for adults.

Measurement of FSH and LH can be done to rule out other causes of anovulation.[8] High FSH indicates primary ovarian failure, low LH indicates hypogonadism, and high LH/FSH ratio is suggestive of PCOS. 17 hydroxyprogesterone levels rule out adrenal hyperplasia, values >200 ng/dL are suggestive of and >1,000 ng/dL are confirmatory of adrenal etiology. Ultrasound is necessary to identify polycystic ovaries and rule out other virilizing tumors that can cause anovulation and hyperandrogenism. Fasting lipid profile, glucose tolerance test are needed to rule out metabolic syndrome and diabetes mellitus. Thyroid profile, prolactin can be done to complete hormonal evaluation of anovulation.

TREATMENT

Symptomatic management aims at addressing menstrual irregularity, clinical hyperandrogenism, and complications of metabolic syndrome. Management of obesity and related comorbidities is by lifestyle modification, diet, and exercise.[9] Weight reduction can improve 50% symptoms of PCOS and normalize hormone levels. Exercise improves sensitivity to insulin and prevents onset of diabetes mellitus.

Metformin can be used as insulin sensitizer in cases of glucose intolerance. Otherwise, it has no role in weight reduction and hence, is no longer used in first-line management of PCOS.

Cyclic hormonal administration in the form of combined oral contraceptive (COC) pills forms first-line management. This COC ensures withdrawal bleeding; thereby, preventing endometrial carcinoma and also inhibits ovarian function and steroidogenesis. These COCs can be withdrawn after 3 months to check for persistent hyperandrogenic anovulation. COC also helps in treating acne and hirsutism in some women. COCs containing cyproterone acetate (Yasmin) help in treating hirsutism with their antiandrogenic action.

In refractory cases, antiandrogens like spironolactone 50–100 mg bd may be used to counter hyperandrogenism. Depilatory creams, waxing, and shaving are also used to remove excess hair. Long-term removal of unwanted hair by laser, electrolysis is more expensive.

Surgical management like ovarian wedge resection, ovarian drilling under laparoscopy have fallen out of favor as treatment options as they compromise the ovarian function. They are used as last resort in some refractory cases to counter stromal hyperplasia and hyperandrogenism. They carry risk of adhesions and decreased ovarian reserve.

Apart from these physical symptoms, PCOS also affects emotional status of the adolescent as they are more prone to body image issues, low self-esteem at this age. This can lead on to depression. Identification, reassurance, and counseling along with medical management improve their quality of life.

CONCLUSION

Polycystic ovary syndrome is a very common condition with severe morbidity affecting quality of life. Early diagnosis and treatment of this condition can prevent the metabolic complications due to this condition.

REFERENCES

1. Vink JM, Sardazeh S, Lambalk CB. Heritability of polycystic ovary syndrome in a Dutch twin family study. J Clin Endocrin Metab. 2006;91(6):2100-4.
2. van Hooff MH, Voorhorst FJ, Kaptein MB, Hirasing RA, Koppenaal C, Schoemaker J. Predictive value of menstrual cycle pattern, body mass index, hormone levels and polycystic ovaries at age 15 years for oligo-amenorrhea at age 18 years. Hum Reprod. 2004;19(2):383-92.
3. Martin KA, Anderson RR, Chang RJ, Ehrmann DA, Lobo RA, Murad MH, et al. Evaluation and treatment of hirsutism in premenopausal women: an endocrine society clinical practice guideline. J Clin Endocrinol Metab. 2018;103(4):1233-57.
4. Kenigsberg LE, Agarwal C, Sin S, Shifteh K, Isasi CR, Crespi R, et al. Clinical utility of magnetic resonance imaging and ultrasonography for diagnosis of polycystic ovary syndrome in adolescent girls. Fertil Steril. 2015;104(5):1302-9.
5. Hart R, Doherty DA. The potential implications of a PCOS diagnosis on a women's long-term health using data linkage. J Clin Endocrinol Metab. 2015;100(3):911-9.
6. Ehrmann DA. Polycystic ovary syndrome. N Eng J Med. 2005;352(12):1223-36.
7. Witchel SF, Oberfield S, Rosenfield RL, Codner E, Bonny A, Ibáñez L, et al. The diagnosis of polycystic ovary syndrome during adolescence. Horm Res Pediatr. 2015;83(6):376-89.
8. Rosenfield RL. Clinical review: adolescent anovulation: maturational mechanisms and implications. J Clin Endocrinol Metab. 2013;98(9):3572-83.
9. Naderpoor N, Shorakae S, de Courten B, Misso ML, Moran LJ, Teede HJ. Metformin and lifestyle modification in polycystic ovary syndrome: systematic review and meta-analysis. Hum Reprod Update. 2015;21(5):560-74.

CHAPTER 3

Primary Amenorrhea

Alok Sharma, Geetika Gupta Syal, Aanya Sharma

INTRODUCTION

Amenorrhea means absence of menstruation.[1] It is more of a symptom than a disease itself. Amenorrhea can be attributed to dysfunction in five compartments which include hypothalamus, pituitary, ovaries, uterus, and vagina, eventually resulting in intermittent, transitory, or permanent cessation of the menstruation. Amenorrhea can be classified as primary and secondary types.

BACKGROUND

The World Health Organization (WHO) defines primary amenorrhea[2] as:
- Absence of menstruation by age 13 years in absence of normal growth or secondary sexual development.
- Absence of menstruation by age 15 years in presence of normal growth and secondary sexual development.

Primary amenorrhea is attributed to a lot of underlying etiologies though majority of which are rare. However, all cases of secondary amenorrhea can also present as primary amenorrhea.

PATHOPHYSIOLOGY OF MENSTRUAL BLEEDING

The circulating estrogen levels in the female circulation initiates the growth and proliferation of the endometrial lining and after ovulation, corpus luteum produces progesterone which transforms the proliferated endometrial lining into secretory endometrium followed by menstruation. The entire menstruation and hormonal milieu are maintained and regulated by the hypothalamic-pituitary-ovarian (HPO) axis.[3] The basic five factors which formulate the synchronized shedding of the endometrium include:
1. Normal female chromosomal patterns
2. Well-coordinated HPO axis
3. Correct and patent anatomy and outflow of the genital tract
4. Well responsive endometrium
5. Active support of the thyroid and adrenal glands.

Any pathophysiological change in the above patterns can be the underlying cause for cessation of menstruation.

CAUSES OF PRIMARY AMENORRHEA[2]

There are many classifications for defining the causes of primary amenorrhea.

The WHO classifies into three classes:
1. *Class 1*: Endogenous estrogen absent, lower normal follicle-stimulating hormone (FSH), and normal prolactin
2. *Class 2*: Normal estrogen, normal FSH, and normal prolactin
3. *Class 3*: High FSH, normal prolactin.

A practical systematic approach which is useful clinically is to group patients on the basis of whether there has been prior estrogen exposure, in which case breasts will be present and whether the uterus is present or absent. *On the basis of physical examination*, the patients can be classified into four groups:
1. Breasts absent, uterus present
2. Breasts present, uterus present
3. Breasts present, uterus absent
4. Breasts absent, uterus absent.

Another Classification on Gonadotropin Levels

Hypergonadotropic Hypogonadism (Primary Amenorrhea)

- *Abnormal sex chromosomes*:
  - *Gonadal dysgenesis*: Turner syndrome (most common cause)
  - Mosaics, abnormal X chromosome.
- *Normal sex chromosomes*:
  - 46,XX pure gonadal dysgenesis
  - 46,XY gonadal dysgenesis—Swyer syndrome

- Gonadotropin-resistant ovary syndrome—Savage syndrome.
- *Enzyme deficiencies*:
  - 17 alpha-hydroxylase deficiency
  - 17, 20-lyase deficiency—aromatase deficiency
  - Congenital lipoid adrenal hyperplasia
  - Galactosemia.

Hypogonadotropic Hypogonadism (Primary Amenorrhea)

- *Hypothalamic causes*:
  - Constitutional delay
  - Gonadotropin-releasing hormone (GnRH) deficiency
  - Hypothalamic hypogonadism (Kallmann syndrome)
  - Psychogenic causes
  - Weight loss, stress
  - Anorexia nervosa
  - Malnutrition.
- *Pituitary causes*:
  - Pituitary hypoplasia—Simmonds disease, pineal gland tumors, and Forbes-Albright syndrome
  - Neoplasms—prolactinomas, craniopharyngiomas, adenomas, and empty sella turcica.
- *Genetic disorders*:
  - 5 alpha-reductase deficiency
  - Gonadotropin-releasing hormone receptor mutation
  - Follicle-stimulating hormone deficiency.

Eugonadotropic Eugonadism (Primary Amenorrhea)

- *Absence of Müllerian development*:
  - Androgen insensitivity syndrome
  - Mayer-Rokitansky-Küster-Hauser syndrome.
- *Normal Müllerian development*:
  - Transverse vaginal septum, imperforate hymen, and female or true intersex
  - Adult-onset congenital adrenal hyperplasia, Cushing disease, thyroid disease, and polycystic ovary syndrome (PCOS).

■ EVALUATION OF PRIMARY AMENORRHEA

When to evaluate?[4]

- No menstruation by the age of 13 years in the absence of growth or development of secondary sexual characteristics.
- No menstruation by the age of 15 years regardless of the presence of normal growth and development of secondary sexual characteristics.
- In women who have menstruated previously, no menses for an interval of time equivalent to total of at least three previous cycles or 6 months.

History

A well-documented history is very essential for analyzing the primary amenorrhea.

- *Development of sexual characters*: Time of appearance, time of menarche, and family history in detail.
- *Symptoms of abdominal pain*: Cyclical pain, duration of onset of pain, type, aggravating factors, and relieving factors (associated with transverse septum, imperforate hymen).
- Any associated difficulty in micturition, dysuria, and urinary retention (hematocolpos).
- History of sexual activity (pregnancy needs to be ruled out prior to establishment of any other diagnosis).
- Any history of virilization (adrenal secreting tumors)
- History of galactorrhea (hyperprolactinoma)
- History of anosmia (Kallmann syndrome)
- History of headache, blurring of vision (pituitary tumor)
- History of abnormal eating patterns
- History of excessive exercises
- History of chronic diseases such as diabetes, tuberculosis, and malnutrition.

Physical Examination

Detailed general physical examination is must in a primary amenorrhea as the genetic disorders have typical physical appearances and play a definite background for establishing further diagnosis.

In the initial evaluation, it is important to determine the presence or absence of the uterus in these patients.

In syndromes like Turner syndrome, features such as low webbed neck, short stature, shielded chest, low lying hair, high-arched palate, and multiple pigmented hairs are few unique features.[5] In Klinefelter syndrome tall habitus is the main feature. Therefore, a detailed general physical examination is important.

Along with above features, detailed system evaluation of all the systems like cardiovascular system, neurological examination and abdominal examination are must to rule out for cardiac lesions, skeleton abnormalities, and renal abnormalities accordingly.[1]

A detailed examination of secondary sexual characters is a necessity in a case of primary amenorrhea. Tanner breast and pubic hair classification help to delineate the management scenario. Discharge from multiple duct—galactorrhea → hyperprolactinemia. Absent or scanty growth of pubic hair as compared to asymmetrically advanced breast development is suggestive of androgen insensitivity syndrome.

Pelvic examination is crucial for all cases of primary amenorrhea and should be performed in the presence of female attendant.

Visual examination helps to identify imperforate hymen if there is a bulging membrane at introitus, transverse vaginal septum can be detected, and absence of patent vagina in Müllerian agenesis. A per rectal examination can be performed to get additional information regarding the uterus.

INVESTIGATIONS

The investigations in a case of primary amenorrhea depend upon presence or absence of secondary sexual characters.

- First step is to rule out physiological amenorrhea which includes baseline investigations like complete hemogram, thyroid function tests, FSH, luteinizing hormone (LH), and serum prolactin levels. Imaging modalities such as ultrasonography (USG) of pelvis and abdomen, chest X-ray can be done. Other special investigations include dehydroepiandrosterone sulfate (DHEAS), free testosterone level, gonadotropin stimulation test, serum cortisol level, oral glucose tolerance test, insulin level, and insulin-like growth factor-1 (IGF-1) according to the need after the history and detailed physical examination **(Table 1)**.
- *Laboratory tests*: Evaluation of FSH and LH.[4]
    - Normal level of FSH and LH—functional ovarian follicles
    - High levels of FSH and LH—reliable indicator of ovarian follicular depletion **(Flowchart 1)**.

To differentiate hypothalamic from pituitary cause of hypogonadotropic amenorrhea, Gonadotropin challenge test is done, where bolus of exogenous GnRH repeated GnRH of 5–10 µg is given at 2–3 hours interval and serum FSH and LH levels are measured; if the levels are low, pituitary cause is established and if they are high, hypothalamic cause is established.

In cases of raised *prolactin levels*, hyperprolactinemia is evaluated for pituitary adenoma. *Serum thyroid-stimulating hormone (TSH)* levels help to differentiate hyperthyroidism and hypothyroidism **(Table 2)**.

Karyotyping is required:

- When the secondary sexual characters are normal but there is absence of uterus where established and in case of presence of the uterus, hermaphrodite (46,XX, 46,XY, and 47,XXY) is to be established.
- In cases of elevated FSH levels.

Ultrasonography of pelvis to confirm the presence or absence of uterus.

CT, MRI for central nervous system (CNS) lesions if galactorrhea, headaches, and/or visual field defects are identified.

X-ray for bone age: In cases to establish constitutional delay.

Before the establishment of treatment with any type of primary amenorrhea, pregnancy should be excluded.

Table 1: Causes of primary amenorrhea according to physical examination.

	Breasts present	Breasts absent
Uterus present	• Hypothalamic • Pituitary • Ovarian • Outflow tract obstruction	• *Primary gonadal failure (high FSH, LH):* – Gonadal dysgenesis syndrome • *CNS hypothalamic pituitary failure (low FSH, LH):* – Idiopathic GnRH deficiency – Constitutional delay
Uterus absent	• Müllerian agenesis • Testicular feminization	• 17,20-desmolase deficiency (46,XX) • 17 alpha-hydroxylase deficiency (46,XY)

(FSH: follicle-stimulating hormone; LH: luteinizing hormone; CNS: central nervous system; GnRH: gonadotropin-releasing hormone)

TREATMENT

The various treatment modalities for primary amenorrhea are individualized according to the classification of primary amenorrhea group.

Hypergonadotropic Hypogonadism (Primary Amenorrhea)

- *Abnormal sex chromosomes*:
    - *Gonadal dysgenesis*: Most common is *Turner syndrome*.[5] Estrogen therapy with 0.25–0.5 mg micronized estradiol increasing gradually at interval of 3–6 months to complete sexual maturation over a period of 2–3 years. And after vaginal bleeding or after 24 months of the therapy, a progesterone should be added to prevent endometrial hyperplasia. Medroxyprogesterone acetate (MPA) can be given either daily in doses of 2.5 mg or cyclically in doses of 5–10 mg for 14 days in a month. Oral micronized

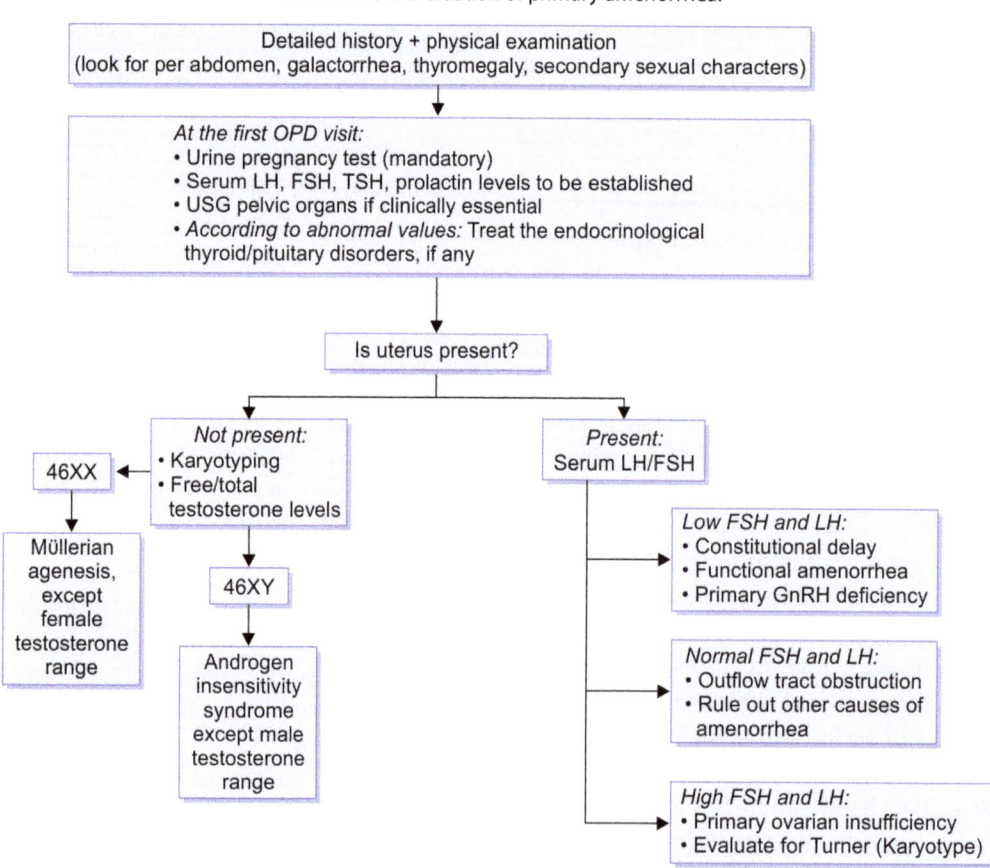

Flowchart 1: Evaluation of primary amenorrhea.

(FSH: follicle-stimulating hormone; GnRH: gonadotropin-releasing hormone; LH: luteinizing hormone; OPD: outpatient department; TSH: thyroid-stimulating hormone; USG: ultrasonography)

progesterone in doses of 100 mg daily or 200 mg for 14 days in a month can also be administered. In case of growth of the female <5th percentile, then growth hormone should be started. Pregnancy is to be avoided in Turner syndrome due to increased chance of aortic dissection. The couple can plan pregnancy by surrogacy.
- *Mosaicism*: 45X/46,XX is the common karyotype seen. In comparison with pure 45X cell line, mosaics are taller and have few abnormalities although 80% are shorter than peers and 66% have somatic abnormalities. Spontaneous menstruation is approximately 20%, but they experience premature menopause because functioning follicles undergo accelerated rate of atresia.
- *Pure gonadal dysgenesis*:
  - *46,XY gonadal dysgenesis*: It indicates bilateral streak ovaries with normal streak ovaries, no chromosomal abnormality, and normal stature.
  - *Swyer syndrome* is the mutation in *SRY* gene. They are XY females with gonadal dysgenesis. Vagina, cervix, and uterus develop normally.

Table 2: Causes of primary amenorrhea according to gonadotrophin levels.

Clinical states	Serum FSH	Serum LH
Normal adult	5–20 IU/L (midcycle peak = 2 × basal level)	5–20 IU/L (midcycle peak = 3 × basal level)
Hypogonadotropic states	<5 IU/L	<5 IU/L
Hypergonadotropic states	>20 IU/L	>40 IU/L

(FSH: follicle-stimulating hormone; LH: luteinizing hormone)

Due to increased malignancy risk around 20–30%, gonadectomy is needed soon after the diagnosis and pregnancy is planned by in vitro fertilization (IVF).
- *Frasier syndrome* is normal female internal and external genitalia, streak gonads, and progressive glomerulopathy. Chance of gonadoblastoma is more common in this category. Gonadectomy is needed for treatment.

46,XX pure gonadal dysgenesis is caused by presence of small Y chromosome fragments in the genome.

In all cases whose karyotype contains Y chromosome, gonadectomy is advised as they are at increased risk of malignant transformation like gonadoblastoma, dysgerminomas, and yolk sac tumors.

- *Enzyme deficiencies*: The various enzyme deficiencies like congenital adrenal deficiencies, 17 alpha-hydroxylase deficiency, and 17 alpha-desmolase deficiency can be treated according to the enzyme deficiencies. Cortisol therapy is the baseline treatment of these treatments.

Hypogonadotropic Hypogonadism (Primary Amenorrhea)

- *Physiological delay*: It is a diagnosis of exclusion. Just reassurance is recommended. Maximum females menstruate with 1–2 years (by 18 years). Pulsatile GnRH is the treatment of choice if needed.
- *Kallmann syndrome*: It is the defective *KAL-1* gene with the failure of migration of olfactory placode leading to failure of GnRH. Treatment is with pulsatile GnRH therapy.
- *Malnutrition, anemia, and anorexia nervosa* counseling is needed with good dietary intake and psychiatric treatment. Some girls may need cyclical estrogens and progesterone therapy. For women desiring pregnancy, ovulation induction can be tried.
- *Hyperprolactinoma* is treated by dopamine agonist therapy by cabergoline or bromocriptine. Macroprolactinoma should be evaluated by the neurosurgical need. MRI of brain and pituitary should be done to rule out CNS tumors.

Eugonadotropic Eugonadism (Primary Amenorrhea)

- *Müllerian anomalies (Mayer-Rokitansky-Küster-Hauser syndrome)*:[6] It is the condition associated with triad of Müllerian agenesis (with absence of vagina, absent uterus, and presence of distal one-third of fallopian tubes), skeletal abnormalities, and renal abnormalities. The sexual secondary characters are normal and ovaries are normal. Vaginoplasty is recommended by methods such as McIndoe procedure and Williams surgery and she cannot become pregnant, but can become mother by surrogacy as they have well-functioning ovaries.
- *Androgen insensitivity syndrome* is the condition where testes and testosterone are present, but testosterone receptors are insensitive with a karyotype of 46,XY with X-linked recessive trait. They are genotypically male, but phenotypically females. Uterus is absent and vagina is with blind ending pouch. They mainly have undescended testis where gonadectomy is very important. After puberty, replacement with cyclical estrogen is needed after puberty. But such phenotypically females can neither have pregnancy nor their own babies and associated with worse reproductive outcome. However, due to more medicolegal issues and awareness among the patients, detailed scenario should be explained to the patient and family members. Proper counseling is also needed.
- *Imperforate hymen:* It is the condition with association of abdominal cyclical pain but no menstruation. Diagnosed generally as blue bulging membranes at introitus and the treatment includes simple cruciate incision. Imperforate hymen is associated with increased risk of endometriosis due to retrograde menstruation.
- *Transverse vaginal septum:* It is due to the fusion disorder of Müllerian duct and urogenital sinuses. Treatment is excision of septum and vaginoplasty.
- *Endocrinological disorders* like PCOS, hypo-, or hyperthyroidism should be treated accordingly.

CONCLUSION

Primary amenorrhea can be attributed to a lot of underlying causes, majority of which are rare. A detailed symptomatic, compartment-based approach will help us to evaluate the causes and to plan a cost effective approach to establish a correct diagnosis. Treatment involves lifelong well-being of the patient along with hormonal replacement, sexual health and fertility.

REFERENCES

1. Practice Committee of the American Society for Reproductive Medicine. Current evaluation of amenorrhea. Fertil Steril. 2006;86:S148-55.
2. Berek JS. Puberty. In: Berek JS (Ed). Berek and Novak's Gynecology, 15th edition. Philadelphia: Lippincott Williams and Wilkins; 2011. pp. 991-1034.
3. Samal R, Habeebullah S. Primary amenorrhea: a clinical review. Int J Reprod Contracept Obstet Gynecol. 2017;6:4748-53.
4. Marc AF, Speroff L. Amenorrhea. In: Taylor HS, Pal L, Sell E (Eds). Speroff's Clinical Gynecologic Endocrinology and Infertility, 9th edition. Philadelphia: Wolters Kluwer (Replica Press); 2015. pp. 435-93.
5. Virginia PS, Elizabeth MC. Turner's Syndrome. N Engl J Med. 2004;351:1227-38.
6. Guerrier D, Mouchel T, Pasquier L, Pellerin I. The Mayer-Rokitansky-Küster-Hauser syndrome (congenital absence of uterus and vagina)—phenotypic manifestations and genetic approaches. J Negat Results Biomed. 2006;5:1.

CHAPTER 4

Congenital Anomalies: Future Fertility!

Shyjus Puliyathinkal

■ INTRODUCTION

When congenital anomalies affected the intrauterine fetus, many a times, the only question that used to be asked was whether it was lethal or not. But these days, with better imaging techniques and rising expectations about the unborn baby, even anomalies affecting the future fertility are being discussed.

The abnormalities in the female baby can be divided based upon the part of the reproductive system affected.

■ ANOMALIES AFFECTING THE UTERUS

Arcuate Uterus

It is identified with a slight midline indentation of the endometrium, at the uterine fundus (**Fig. 1**). It is a normal variant and does not affect future fertility.[1]

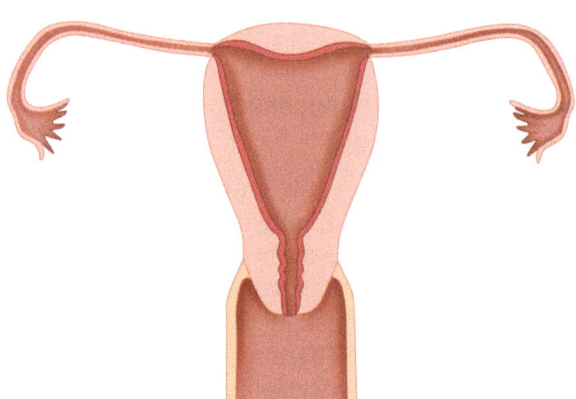

Fig. 1: Arcuate uterus.

Septate or Subseptate Uterus

The septate uterus (**Fig. 2**) is the most common uterine anomaly. A defect in canalization of the two fused Müllerian ducts or a defect in resorption of its midline septum results in this condition. The degree of septation varies widely from a partial midline septum (a subseptate uterus) with one cervix to complete failure of resorption resulting in a longitudinal septum that begins from the fundus into the vagina.

Ultrasound findings of two closely separated endometrial cavities and a smooth fundal contour establishes the diagnosis. The depth from the interstitial line to the apex of the indentation is greater than 1.5 cm, and the angle of indentation is less than 90°. The diagnosis is either done with a 3D ultrasound or an magnetic resonance imaging (MRI). The sensitivity and specificity of MRI for diagnosis of septate uterus is as high as 100% since it clearly shows whether the fundal contour is smooth or indented.

Women with septate uterus are at increased risk for spontaneous abortion (20–40%) and preterm delivery

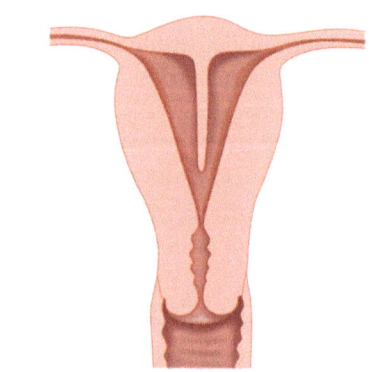

Fig. 2: Septate uterus.

(10–30%). The live birth rate ranges from 50 to 70%. The septate uterus is also associated with an increased risk of breech presentation and abruption.

Resection of the septum hysteroscopically (hysteroscopic metroplasty) can improve pregnancy outcome.[2]

Bicornuate Uterus

A bicornuate uterus (**Fig. 3**) has a fundal indentation >1 cm, with the vagina and cervix being generally normal. It results from partial fusion of the Müllerian ducts. Depending on

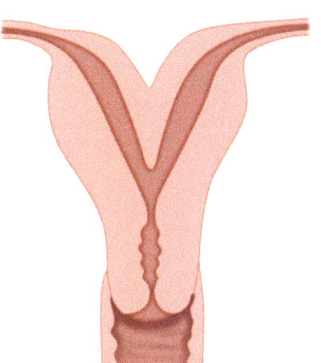

Fig. 3: Bicornuate uterus.

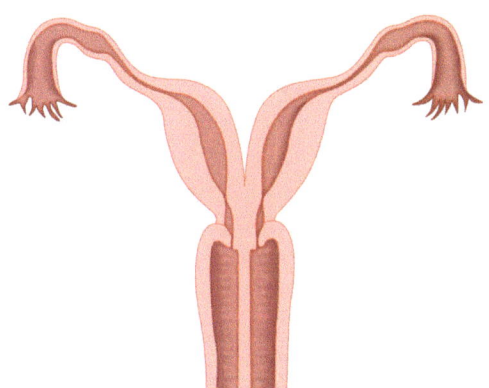

Fig. 4: Uterus didelphys.

the extent of fusion, separation of the uterine horns will be complete, partial or minimal.

Two moderately separated endometrial cavities and an indented fundal contour establishes the diagnosis in ultrasound. 3D ultrasonography can reliably differentiate between septate and bicornuate uteri by simultaneously visualizing both the external and internal contours of the uterine fundus. MRI is rarely needed to make a definitive diagnosis and should be reserved for times when 3D ultrasonography is not available or the results are inconclusive, or in cases with suspected complex anomalies involving multiple systems.[3]

Spontaneous abortion in 36%, preterm birth in 21-23%, and fetal survival in 50-60% of patients with a bicornuate uterus, is what the data tells us. Fetal growth restriction and malpresentation in labor are also increased.

In patients with poor pregnancy outcomes that are thought to be related to the anomaly, uterine reunification can be performed via laparotomy. Due to an association between bicornuate uterus and cervical insufficiency, the cervical length should be assessed during pregnancy.

Uterus Didelphys

It is a duplication of reproductive structures. Generally, the duplication is limited to the uterus and cervix [uterine didelphys and bicollis (two cervices)], although duplication of the vulva, bladder, urethra, vagina, and anus may also occur. Uterine didelphys **(Fig. 4)** occurs when the two Müllerian ducts fail to fuse. About 15-20% of women with didelphic uterus also have unilateral anomalies, such as an obstructed hemivagina and ipsilateral renal agenesis.

Ultrasound shows two widely separated uterine horns with a deep fundal indentation and speculum examination shows two cervixes. MRI is rarely needed to make a definitive diagnosis. Spontaneous abortion rates of 32% and preterm birth rates of 28% have been noted. Fetal growth restriction also appears to be increased. A septated vagina is an association and may cause difficulty with sexual intercourse or vaginal delivery. Metroplasty should be considered for women with pelvic pain, recurrent miscarriages, or a history of preterm delivery. Women with an obstructed hemivagina and ipsilateral renal agenesis will have regular menses because menstrual blood from one uterus can come out through its nonobstructed cervix and hemivagina. However, such patients will most likely develop cyclic pain due to buildup of blood in the obstructed hemivagina. In addition, there may be a micro-communication between the patent vagina and the obstructed vagina, resulting in an infected obstructed hemivagina. Treatment involves resection of the wall of the obstructed vagina followed by creation of a single vaginal vault.

Unicornuate Uterus

In the unicornuate uterus **(Figs. 5A to D)**, one cavity is usually normal, with a Fallopian tube and cervix, while the failed Müllerian duct takes various forms. The affected Müllerian duct may not develop at all, or it may develop only partially as either a rudimentary horn or an anlage (a cluster of embryonic cells). This horn may or may not communicate with the uterus.

Diagnosis is made by ultrasound, showing a uterus deviated to one side of the pelvis. Care should be taken to assess the presence of a rudimentary horn. In complicated cases where surgical removal is being considered for a rudimentary horn, MRI can be helpful in surgical planning.

Most rudimentary horns are asymptomatic. Some contain functional endometrium that gets shed cyclically. If a rudimentary horn is obstructed, the woman may develop cyclic or chronic abdomino-pelvic pain and may require surgical excision of the obstructed horn.

Women with a unicornuate uterus are at higher risk for endometriosis, preterm labor, and breech presentation.

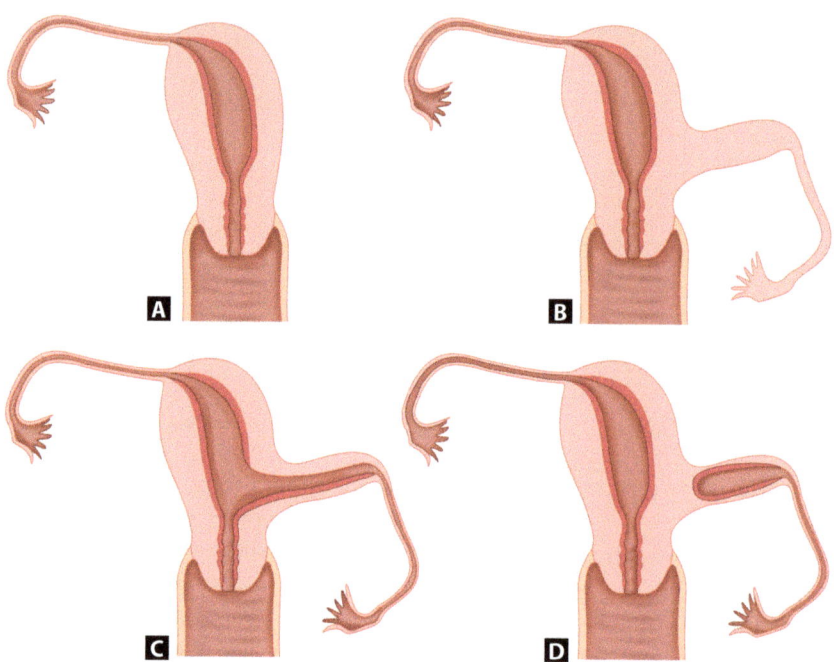

Figs. 5A to D: *Unicornuate uterus subtypes*: (A) Unicornuate uterus with no rudimentary horn; (B) A rudimentary horn without a uterine cavity; (C) A rudimentary horn with a communicating cavity to the normal side; (D) A rudimentary horn with a non-communicating cavity.

Rates of obstetric complications are: 2.7% ectopic pregnancy, 24% first-trimester abortion, 10% second-trimester abortion, 20% preterm delivery, 4% fetal demise, and 50% live births.[4]

Uterine rupture and/or adherent placental abnormalities are associated with pregnancies in an obstructed or rudimentary uterine horn. Thus, such pregnancies should be immediately terminated. Unicornuate uterus is associated with a particularly high incidence (40%) of renal abnormalities.

Women with unicornuate uteri are generally not candidates for reconstructive procedures to improve pregnancy outcome, given that this anomaly is associated with generally favorable pregnancy outcomes.[5] However, a rudimentary horn with functioning endometrium can harbor an ectopic pregnancy, and thus noncommunicating rudimentary horns with endometrium may, at times, be surgically removed.

■ ANOMALIES OF HYMEN

Hymenal anomalies are derived from incomplete degeneration of the central part of the hymen.

Imperforate Hymen

It is one of the most common obstructive lesions of the female genital tract. In neonates, the diagnosis is made, if a bulging introitus is noted at birth. The bulging is due to a mucocolpos from vaginal secretions due to stimulation by maternal estradiol. If the diagnosis is not made in the newborn period and the hymen remains imperforate, the mucus will be reabsorbed and the child usually remains asymptomatic until menarche.

At the expected age of menarche, the adolescent girl may present with amenorrhea (sometimes referred to as crypto-menarche), cyclic abdominal or pelvic pain, and hematocolpos, which may give the hymenal membrane a bluish discoloration. Marked distension of the vagina may also result in back pain, pain with defecation or difficulties with urination.

There is typically a bulging obstruction of the vagina. It is important that the clinician does not assume that all bulging obstructive anomalies of the vagina are an imperforate hymen. The differential diagnosis includes agenesis of the lower vagina or a low transverse vaginal septum.

The diagnosis can be confirmed with the use of a translabial or transabdominal ultrasound to determine the distance from the obstruction to the level of the normal location of an introitus. If there is a thin structure (few millimeters) obstructing the introitus, then it is most likely the membrane of an imperforate hymen. But if obstructing structure is thicker, the diagnosis is not an imperforate hymen.

Treatment

Repair of an imperforate hymen can be performed at any age; however, the repair is facilitated if the tissues have undergone estrogen stimulation. Therefore, surgery is ideal in the neonatal period or postpubertal/premenarchal period. Surgical repair, performed under anesthesia, consists of an elliptical incision in the membrane close to the hymenal ring followed by evacuation of the obstructed material. Extra-hymenal tissue is excised using electrocautery to create a normal size orifice and the vaginal mucosa is sutured to the hymenal ring using 3-0 or 4-0 vicryl or chromic suture to prevent adhesion and recurrence of the obstruction **(Fig. 6)**.

A simple incision and drainage is not adequate treatment as it may not permit complete egress of the built up menstrual blood and may lead to an ascending infection due to ascending bacteria infecting the remaining blood in the vagina, uterus, and/or fallopian tubes.

■ ANOMALIES OF THE VAGINA

Transverse Vaginal Septum

It results when there is failure of fusion and/or canalization of the urogenital sinus and Müllerian ducts. The septa are generally less than 1 cm in thickness, tend to have a fenestration and thus, are not completely obstructed. Children may present with mucocolpos, whereas adolescents may develop a mucocolpos, hematocolpos or pyohematocolpos due to an ascending infection through the small perforation.

Ultrasonographic imaging helps to define the location and thickness of the septum and the distance from the obstructing tissue to the level of the introitus **(Fig. 7)**. Ultrasound or MRI can be helpful to differentiate between a high septum versus congenital absence of the cervix.

For treatment, a small, thin septum can be primarily resected, followed by an end-to-end anastomosis of the upper and lower vaginal mucosa.

A thick septum is more difficult to excise and repair and has a higher risk of restenosis and obstruction. Primary anastomosis is easier if the upper vagina has been distended with menstrual blood products, as this acts as a natural tissue expander to increase the amount of upper vaginal tissue available for the anastomosis. In the postoperative period, patients need teaching on how to utilize vaginal dilators to assist with healing and avoid scar tissue formation and stenosis.

Longitudinal Vaginal Septum

These are typically associated with uterine anomalies, such as septate uterus and uterus didelphys. On physical examination, a longitudinal vaginal septum **(Fig. 8)** will be visualized as a fibrous structure dividing the vagina in

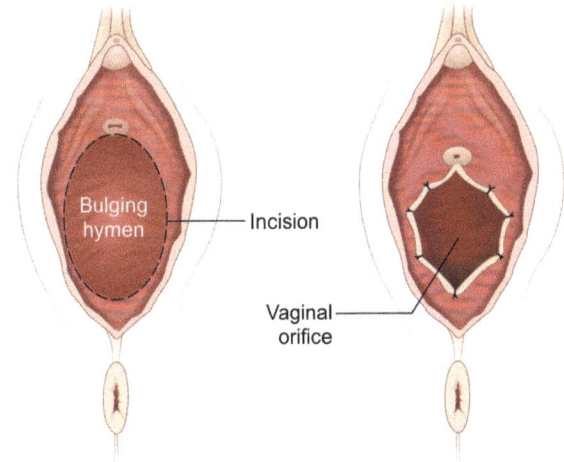

Fig. 6: Incision in surgical repair for imperforate hymen.

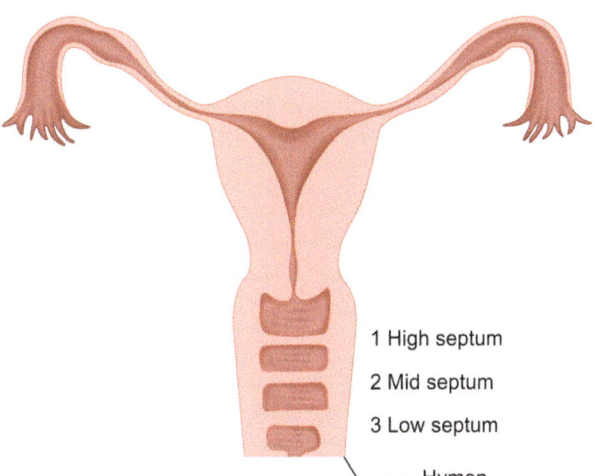

Fig. 7: Types of transverse vaginal septum.

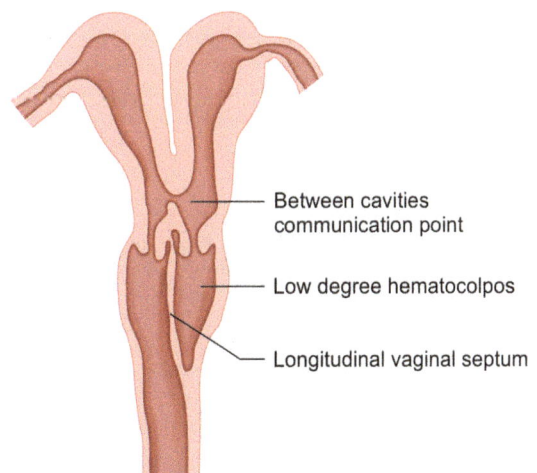

Fig. 8: Longitudinal vaginal septum with uterus didelphys.

half. Imaging should determine if there is a single cervix or two cervixes with one at the apex of each vagina. This can be accomplished with two-dimensional ultrasound, three-dimensional ultrasound, or MRI. Surgery is not required in asymptomatic women with a longitudinal vaginal septum, but will facilitate vaginal delivery.

Treatment involves complete resection of the septum, with care to avoid compromise to the bladder and rectum. The septal tissue is resected by wedging out the fibrous septum, and then the normal mucosa from each vagina is sutured together over the defect created by the resection.

Vaginal Agenesis

Also known as Müllerian agenesis or Mayer-Rokitansky-Küster-Hauser (MRKH) syndrome **(Fig. 9)**, it refers to the congenital absence of the vagina with variable uterine development. It results from agenesis or hypoplasia of the Müllerian duct system, although the underlying etiology remains unknown. A genetic analysis of MRKH syndrome in a large cohort of families showed that the prevalence of *WNT3, HNF1B, and LHX1* point mutations is low in people with MRKH.

It is usually accompanied by cervical and uterine agenesis; however, 7-10% of women have functional endometrium within either a uterus that is obstructed, but otherwise structurally normal. Ovaries were normal in 78% of affected patients, 16% had extra-pelvic ovaries, and 6% had unilateral hypoplastic ovaries.[6] Rates of associated renal comorbidities have varied from 5 to 34%.

Approximately, 25-50% have urologic anomalies, such as unilateral renal agenesis, pelvic or horseshoe kidneys, or irregularities of the collecting system, and 10-15% have skeletal anomalies involving the spine, ribs, and extremities.[7] Other less common anomalies include congenital heart lesions, abnormalities of the hand, deafness, cleft palate, and inguinal or femoral hernias.

Clinical Presentation

Patients with MRKH have a normal female karyotype with normal ovaries and ovarian function, thus they develop normal secondary sexual characteristics (e.g., breast development, axillary hair, and public hair). They often present with primary amenorrhea at 15-17 years of age. Most patients have a rudimentary nonfunctioning uterus, but 2-7% have a uterus with functioning endometrium and may present with cyclic or chronic abdominopelvic pain secondary to hematocolpos, hematometra, hematosalpinx, or endometriosis.

On physical examination, the external genitalia are normal. A vaginal "dimple" or small pouch is typically seen and the hymenal tissue is usually present. Rectoabdominal examination is helpful to determine the presence or absence of the vagina, cervix, and uterus.

Ultrasound examination is performed to assess the kidneys and confirm the presence of ovaries and whether a uterus is present. Possible ureteral duplication can be determined by intravenous pyelography, if indicated. If the patient has pain and the ultrasound shows hemi-uteri without an endometrial stripe, then MRI may be useful for determining whether functional endometrium is present.

Differential diagnosis of vaginal agenesis includes androgen insensitivity, low-lying transverse vaginal septum, agenesis/atresia of the uterus and vagina, and imperforate hymen. First-line treatment for vaginal agenesis is nonsurgical, with use of vaginal dilators. This is highly successful with excellent patient satisfaction.

Surgery may be appropriate if nonsurgical therapy fails or, if after extensive counseling, a patient elects a surgical approach.

Historically, the most commonly performed surgery by gynecologists was the McIndoe vaginoplasty and data from over 1,200 patients show a high success rate (92%).[8] Less invasive laparoscopic surgery, as in the modified Vecchietti or Davydov procedures, is now a more widely accepted option; however, more data about results and long-term complications are needed. Ultimately, the best surgical option is dependent upon the experience of the attending surgeon and the woman's preference based upon the advantages and disadvantages of each procedure. Each procedure has advantages and disadvantages, and there is no "perfect" option.

- The McIndoe procedure, which is often used by gynecologists, utilizes a split-thickness skin graft from

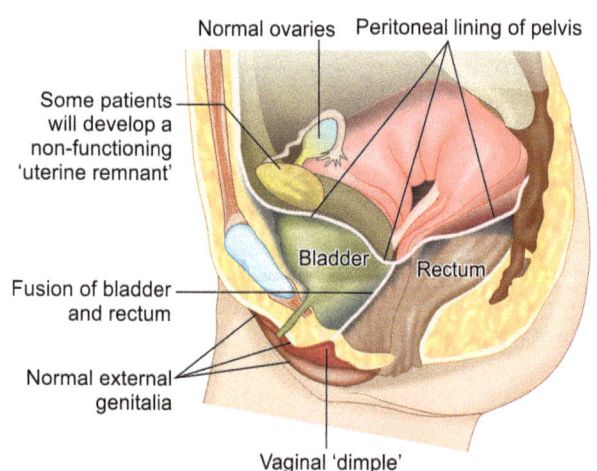

Fig. 9: Mayer–Rokitansky–Küster–Hauser syndrome.

the buttocks. A transverse incision is made at the vaginal dimple and a cavity is dissected to the level of the peritoneum. The mold and skin graft are then inserted, and the labia minora are secured around the stent to prevent expulsion. Postoperatively, a vaginal dilator must be used continuously for 3 months and then at night for 6 additional months to prevent contraction of the vagina.[9]

- The Williams vulvovaginoplasty involves the creation of a vaginal pouch. A horseshoe-shaped incision is made on the perineum and full-thickness skin flaps from the labia majora are used to create a kangaroo-like pouch, which is horizontal to the perineum. A vaginal dilator is then used daily for 3–4 weeks postoperatively.
- Sigmoid vaginoplasty utilizes a segment of sigmoid colon for vaginoplasty. One end of the resected segment is pulled down to the introitus to form a neovagina, and the other end is closed to create a blind pouch. An end-to-end reanastomosis is performed to recreate a patent gastrointestinal tract.
- Vecchietti or modified Vecchietti procedure involves creation of a neovagina by invagination using an acrylic "olive" that is placed against the vaginal dimple. This olive is attached to a traction device that rests on the abdomen by subperitoneal sutures placed laparoscopically. Sufficient traction is applied to the olive to produce 1.0–1.5 cm of invagination per day, thereby creating a neovagina in approximately 7–9 days. Once the neovagina has been created, active dilation is required until regular sexual activity is initiated.
- Davydov procedure is a three stage surgery that includes dissection of the rectovesical space, abdominal mobilization of the peritoneum to create the vaginal fornices, and attachment of the peritoneum to the introitus.

Treatment involves a combination of psychosocial support and correction of the anatomic abnormality.

The psychologic aspects of a new diagnosis of vaginal agenesis can be overwhelming for any patient, especially an adolescent. Emotional support, counseling, and psychological preparation before treatment play critical roles in the resolution of this condition.

A normal sex life is possible after creation of a neovagina. Although, the patient will be unable to carry a pregnancy, her eggs may be harvested for achieving pregnancy with a gestational carrier. Another option is that of uterine transplantation.

REFERENCES

1. Prior M, Richardson A, Asif S, Polanski L, Parris-Larkin M, Chandler J, et al. Outcome of assisted reproduction in women with congenital uterine anomalies: a prospective observational study. Ultrasound Obstet Gynecol. 2018;51(1):110-7.
2. Fedele L, Bianchi S. Hysteroscopic metroplasty for septate uterus. Obstet Gynecol Clin North Am. 1995;22:473-89.
3. Bermejo C, Martínez Ten P, Cantarero R, Diaz D, Pérez Pedregosa J, Barrón E, et al. Three-dimensional ultrasound in the diagnosis of Müllerian duct anomalies and concordance with magnetic resonance imaging. Ultrasound Obstet Gynecol. 2010;35(5):593-601.
4. Reichman D, Laufer MR, Robinson BK. Pregnancy outcomes in unicornuate uteri: a review. Fertil Steril. 2009;91:1886-94.
5. Acién P, Acién M, Sánchez-Ferrer M. Complex malformations of the female genital tract. New types and revision of classification. Hum Reprod. 2004;19:2377-84.
6. Haddad B, Louis-Sylvestre C, Poitout P, Paniel BJ. Longitudinal vaginal septum: a retrospective study of 202 cases. Eur J Obstet Gynecol Reprod Biol. 1997;74(2):197-9.
7. Scanlan KA, Pozniak MA, Fagerholm M, Shapiro S. Value of transperineal sonography in the assessment of vaginal atresia. Am J Roentgenol. 1990;154:545-8.
8. Wu MH, Hsu CC, Huang KE. Detection of congenital müllerian duct anomalies using three-dimensional ultrasound. J Clin Ultrasound. 1997;25:487-92.
9. Jayasinghe Y, Rane A, Stalewski H, Grover S. The presentation and early diagnosis of the rudimentary uterine horn. Obstet Gynecol. 2005;105:1456-67.

CHAPTER 5

Fertility Preservation in Ovarian Tumors in Adolescents

Tripti Sharan, Keerti Khetan

INTRODUCTION

Gynecological cancers are relatively frequent in the female population. Among all ovarian cancers (OCs), 12% are diagnosed in fertile women. OCs account for 1–2% of all pediatric cancer in the age group of 1–15 years.

The incidence of ovarian masses in childhood is 2.6 cases per 100,000 girls per year, of which 50% are malignant, 85% of them are germ cell tumors (GCTs), 8% are epithelial cell carcinoma, and 5% are sex cord stromal tumors.

This population is faced with difficult considerations such as:
- Cancer diagnosis and prognosis
- Treatment options
- Future childbearing potentials.

The overall 5-year survival rate for OCs in women ≤44 years of age is 91.2% at stages 1A and 1B.

Owing to increased survival, there is a new focus on the quality of life (QoL) for cancer patients. Women unable to conceive after cancer treatment experience significant regret so the focus in gynecological cancer treatment especially among young adolescents has shifted toward fertility preservation and also ovarian functions, wherever possible.

For women with OC, it gets more difficult to maintain reproductive function because the ovary is the site of primary cancer.

The challenges in fertility-sparing strategies in this age group are:
- Conserving fertility
- Achieving the longest remission period
- Balancing the therapeutic doses and side effects of cytotoxic drugs.

FERTILITY-SPARING METHODS

For the postpubertal to premenopausal women, ovarian stimulation followed by cryopreservation of embryos or oocytes is the most well-established form of fertility preservation.

Embryo Cryopreservation

Since it was performed for the first time in 1983, embryo cryopreservation has become a proven method of fertility preservation. It is not particularly helpful in adolescents as it requires the presence of a male partner. The ovarian stimulation for retrieval of oocytes has to be started before the chemotherapy is commenced because of poor ovarian response thereafter. It should be possible to defer cancer treatment for at least 2–4 weeks giving time to carry out ovarian stimulation and oocyte retrieval.

Oocyte Cryopreservation

Oocyte cryopreservation is a very good option for patients with unilateral OC. Oocytes could be acquired during unilateral ovariectomy. Controlled ovarian hyperstimulation (COH) is not indicated in case of early intervention or in prepubescent patients and it is also not indicated in patients with granulosa cancer due to rapid hormone-dependent proliferation. The oocytes can be acquired immature or mature.

Immature oocytes are acquired without the need of stimulation and subsequently are matured *in vitro* either before freezing or after thawing. Immature oocytes are more resistant to cryoinjury than mature oocytes since they do not contain a metaphase spindle. Compared to embryo cryopreservation, oocyte freezing is still associated with lower pregnancy rates (4.6–12% vs. 30–40%). Mature oocyte cryopreservation is a strategy for fertility preservation in postpubertal females without a committed male partner and who do not wish to use the donor sperm.

Ovarian Cryopreservation

Ovarian cryopreservation followed by heterotopic implantation or orthotopic implantation is a technique that can be offered to postpubertal women in whom ovarian stimulation is contraindicated or for those in whom cancer treatment cannot be postponed and also those who have hormone-sensitive tumors. It is also the only solution to offer to prepubertal patients. Thawing and regrafting the original cryopreserved tissue could run the risk of reintroducing any malignancy.

Oophoropexy or Ovarian Transposition

This is an option in young women planning pelvic radiation. It involves transposing the ovaries above the pelvic brim and as lateral as possible. Various locations include the base of the round ligament, retroperitoneally on the psoas muscle, at the level of the lower kidney pole, in the paracolic gutters, or transposing the ovaries >1.5 cm above the iliac crest. It could be done laparoscopically unless the patient is already undergoing laparotomy for their primary cancer treatment.

■ FERTILITY PRESERVATION ALONG WITH CHEMOTHERAPY AND RADIOTHERAPY

Surgery is not the only procedure that damages fertility in women with OC. Both chemotherapy and radiation therapy have a harmful effect.

Alkylating agents such as cyclophosphamide are gonadotoxic and have been associated with ovarian failure in a dose-dependent manner. The American Society of Clinical Oncology and Clinical Practice Guidelines Committee stated that women treated with high doses (≥ 5 g/m^2) of alkylating agents have a high risk (>70%) to developing permanent amenorrhea. Alkylating agents determine oocytes damage via single-stranded deoxyribonucleic acid (DNA) breaks and targets cells at every stage of cell cycle, preferentially on primordial follicles. The impact on fertility of taxanes and platinums [most effective for epithelial ovarian cancer (EOC)] is an intermediate risk level (30–70%) of amenorrhea whereas antimetabolites and anthracyclines carry a lower risk (<30%).

Radiation is reserved for chemotherapy-resistant OCs. It has been seen that lower doses of radiation therapy used for OCs resulted in germ cell death in the contralateral ovary in the case of unilateral oophorectomy. Germ cells are the most sensitive cells in the body to radiation and chemotherapy and can be protected from the off-target effects of radiation and chemotherapy through fertiprotective agents.

Fertiprotective Agents

Although cryopreservation methods are effective for fertility conservation, they do not protect ovarian function. Prevention of chemotherapy-associated ovarian failure (COF) reduces the long-term health sequelae of ovarian failure. Therefore, fertility preservation and prevention of COF should occur concurrently.

Gonadotropin-releasing hormone (GnRH) analogs (GnRHa) should be considered in conjunction with cryopreservation to prevent COF. GnRHa protects ovarian function by decreasing ovarian perfusion, decreasing exposure of the primordial follicles to the cytotoxic agents, and may upregulate antiapoptotic molecules. Starting GnRHa at least 1 week before chemotherapy and then continuing throughout chemotherapy can substantially reduce COF and later give higher pregnancy rates. With its ready availability, GnRHa forms an important part in improving survivorship for many young women diagnosed with cancer.

The efficacy of GnRH antagonists in the prevention of COF has been less investigated. Unlike GnRHa, where there is an initial surge in follicle-stimulating hormone (FSH) and luteinizing hormone (LH), GnRH antagonists result in immediate suppression of gonadotropins. This may be advantageous when chemotherapy is required urgently. The combination of GnRHa and GnRH antagonist has been shown to provide suppression of gonadotropin secretion within 96 hours, allowing chemotherapy without delay.

■ PREDICTING OVARIAN RESERVE

Serum anti-Müllerian hormone (AMH) level seems to be the most sensitive measure of ovarian reserve in cancer survivors. It is helpful in determining fertility preservation strategies and anticipating the need for a hormone-based therapy for menopausal symptoms and bone health.

For young ovarian germ cell tumor survivors who have significant reproductive and sexual functioning concerns, problem-solving education and therapy may be beneficial.

■ FERTILITY-SPARING SURGERY

The choice to perform fertility-sparing surgery must take into account the type of tumor and the stage of the disease. The fertility preservation strategies according to the histological type of ovarian tumor are as follows:

- *Germ cell tumors:* Malignant ovarian germ cell tumors (MOGCTs) are rare cancers (3–5% of ovarian tumors), but they are the ones that mostly affect younger women. 83% of cases occur in women under the age of 40 years, often in women in their teens and twenties.

  Approximately 60–70% of cases are diagnosed at FIGO stage I or II, 20–30% are stage III and stage IV and bilateral involvement is relatively uncommon, except in the case of dysgerminomas (10–15%). (FIGO stands for International Federation of Gynecology and Obstetrics) Preservation of fertility is an important aspect in these neoplasms. Because of rapid growth and early symptoms, the tumor is commonly diagnosed in stage I unlike EOC. Unilateral salpingo-oophorectomy with peritoneal staging and retroperitoneal staging if indicated, is the treatment of choice in early stage MOGCT. Careful abdominal exploration with inspection and palpation of all peritoneal surfaces, multiple biopsies of peritoneum and omentectomy should be performed during surgery. There is no survival difference between unilateral or bilateral salpingo-oophorectomy when MOGCT is confined to one ovary. Bilateral disease is uncommon and no biopsy is advised owing to the risk of extra adhesions and impairment of ovarian reserve unless there are macroscopically suspicious areas in the contralateral ovary.

In advanced-stage MOGCTs, neoadjuvant chemotherapy has been used to increase the chance of fertility-preserving surgery, minimizing the extent of surgery required to achieve maximal cytoreduction. Cisplatin-based combination chemotherapy with bleomycin, etoposide, and cisplatin (BEP regimen) is the gold-standard regimen for the first-line treatment of germ cell tumors at all stages.

Cure rates with early-stage MOGCTs approach 100% and even in advanced-stage disease, cure rates are at least 75%.

Although ovarian surgery, radiotherapy, and chemotherapy could compromise ovarian function and fertility, the infertility rate among women attempting conception after treatment for MOGCTs ranges from 5 to 10%, corresponding to the incidence rate of infertility in the normal population.

- *Pure dysgerminoma*: Fertility-sparing treatment is suggested for all stages with a disease-free survival in 10 years of >90% and overall survival 100%. Radiotherapy is the traditional postoperative treatment for patients with dysgerminoma with excellent outcomes.
- *Yolk sac tumors (YSTs) (Nondysgerminomatous tumors)*: For early stages, fertility-sparing surgery is feasible. In higher stages, standard-dose BEP chemotherapy following fertility-sparing surgery has been associated with favorable overall survival rates and no apparent compromise of fertility rates. Serum alpha-fetoprotein (AFP) is a reliable marker for diagnosis and may be used in clinical decision-making after surgery and disease management. Even though three courses of BEP are the standard adjuvant therapy after conservative surgery for early-stage YST, some patients can also be carefully followed up without treatment if AFP after surgery declines consistently.
- *Immature ovarian teratoma (nondysgerminomatous tumors) stage 1 grades 2–3*: Adjuvant chemotherapy following fertility-sparing surgery has been recommended by some, but several studies suggest an expectant approach with BEP only in case of relapse. More than 80% of patients retain reproductive function after chemotherapy and surgery. Oocyte cryopreservation could be proposed to all adolescent patients and to those who have not yet planned a pregnancy.

- *Malignant sex cord stromal tumors*: These tumors are rare and include granulosa cell tumors (most common) and Sertoli-Leydig cell tumors. They have a good prognosis and most present with early-stage disease. Patients with stage IA or IC sex cord stromal tumors can be treated with fertility-sparing surgery. Although complete staging is recommended, lymphadenectomy may be omitted for stage IA or IC. Completion surgery should be considered after childbearing is finished. For patients with high-risk stage I tumors (tumor rupture, stage IC, poorly differentiated tumor, and tumor size >10–15 cm), observation or platinum-based chemotherapy should be indicated. Patients with surgical findings of low-risk stage I tumor (i.e., without high-risk features) should be observed.
- *Borderline tumors*: Borderline ovarian tumors (BOTs) comprise 10–20% of ovarian epithelial tumors and are typically diagnosed during reproductive years. Survival rates are about 99% with a 70-month disease-free survival in cases of stage I tumors and the survival rate in cases of stage III tumors is about 89%. While conventionally bilateral salpingo-oophorectomy has been advocated as the initial treatment for early-stage BOT, studies have reported excellent results with more conservative treatments including cystectomy or unilateral salpingo-oophorectomy. Ovarian corticectomy has also been used for conserving fertility. Fertility-sparing surgery is associated with a higher risk of relapse, but not with increased mortality.

Factors associated with a higher risk of relapse after conservative surgery for early-stage BOT include age < 30 years, bilateral tumor, and type of surgery (cystectomy vs. adnexectomy). Micropapillary histologic pattern, stage, and presence of invasive implants are other well-recognized risk factors. It is best to start planning pregnancy after 3 months from surgery. In adolescents or in those who want to postpone pregnancy, oocyte cryopreservation after ovarian stimulation is advised. Most recurrences were BOT and were successfully managed by surgery.

- *Epithelial tumors*: Although the vast majority of EOC are diagnosed in postmenopausal women and at an advanced stage, 3–17% of EOC occurs in women under 40 years old and only 3–4% in patients under 30 years. The 5-year overall survival rate for young patients with early-stage EOC is generally good ranging between 94 and 98%.

The standard treatment for patients in FIGO stages I-II EOC is total hysterectomy, bilateral salpingo-oophorectomy, peritoneal sampling, omentectomy, and both pelvic and para-aortic lymphadenectomy. According to the available guidelines, in young women, conservative surgery can be performed for all grades at stage IA or IC while this approach is still debated for high-risk patients (clear cell, stage more than or equal to IAG3). In the recent European Society for Medical Oncology (ESMO) and European Society of Gynaecological Oncology (ESGO) guidelines, a conservative approach is limited to G1-2 IA and IC EOC with unilateral involvement in the case of mucinous, serous, endometrioid, or mixed histotype.

The laparoscopic approach is feasible, but tumors >10 cm are at a higher risk of rupture and spillage, 88% versus 9% through laparoscopy compared to laparotomy. Most relapses occurring after a conservative surgery are extraovarian suggesting that the preservation of one ovary is not necessarily the cause of the recurrence. Moreover, the adjuvant therapy in early-stage EOC improves survival and delays recurrence in patients with IC stage.

BRCA Mutation

For healthy BRCA-mutated patients with elevated risk for OC, fertility is affected by treatments of eventual cancer and prevention strategies. The carriers should complete childbearing and undergo a salpingo-oophorectomy around 35–40 years if *BRCA1* mutated and 45–50 years if *BRCA2* mutated while concurrent hysterectomy is not recommended. Those carrying BRCA mutations, especially *BRCA1*, are associated with decreased ovarian reserve leading to infertility and early menopause.

In cases needing fertility preservation, oocyte cryopreservation could be an option for BRCA-mutated women who undergo early surgery. Ovarian tissue cryopreservation is not recommended because of increased risk of malignant transformation.

Salpingectomy with delayed oophorectomy, preserving natural follicular cycle, is another option, but still not recommended as the primary approach.

Carcinosarcomas

Carcinosarcomas malignant mixed Müllerian tumors (MMMTs) are rare tumors with a poor prognosis. Patients with MMMTs are not candidates for fertility-sparing surgery regardless of age.

To sum up, different approaches for each type of tumor are summarized in **Flowchart 1**.

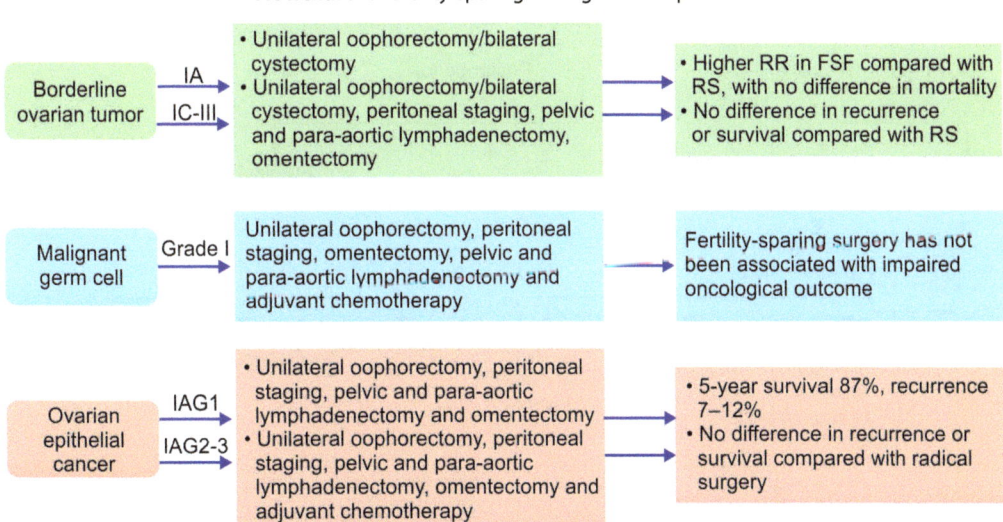

Flowchart 1: Fertility-sparing strategies in OC patients.

(FSF: fertility-sparing surgery; OC: ovarian cancer; RR: recurrence rate; RS: radical surgery)
(*Source:* Adapted from Tomao F, Di Pinto A, Sassu CM, Bardhi E, Di Donato V, Muzii L, et al. Fertility preservation in ovarian tumours. Ecancer Medical Science. 2018;12:885).

FUTURE PERSPECTIVES

Artificial Ovary

Important steps in the development of an artificial ovary have been successfully completed. Researchers reported at the European Society of Human Reproduction and Embryology (ESHRE)-2018 meeting that they have isolated and grown human follicles to a point of biofunctionality on a bioengineered ovarian scaffold made of decellularized ovarian tissue.

In Vitro Ovarian Follicle Growth

The greatest risk associated with cryopreserved ovarian tissue autotransplantation is the possibility of a tumor reimplantation and dissemination, also in the contralateral ovary transplantation that could also contain tumor cells. *In vitro* follicles could represent a chance to preserve fertility in young patients with OC. This technique does not require hormonal stimulation and can also be offered in prepubertal patients.

In Vitro Ovarian Follicle Maturation

A future possibility to offer to young cancer patients could be follicular maturation *in vitro*. A portion of cortical ovarian cysts from patients with cancer could be treated with phosphatase and tensin homolog inhibitor or AKT activator determining *in vitro* ovarian follicle maturation. These follicles can be kept for future use.

Protection against Germ Cell Damage using Fertoprotective Agents

Fertility-sparing surgical approaches have limitations including cost, time, accessibility to dedicated centers, and gonadotoxicity related to procedures. Therefore, the need arises to obtain adjuvants that protect the pool of dormant follicles from the anticancer drugs.

Molecules studied for this role are sphingosine-1-phosphate (S1P), imatinib mesylate, amifostine, tamoxifen, and GnRH antagonists and agonists. There are emerging studies on the fertoprotective role of melatonin. In fact, melatonin reduces the adverse effects of chemotherapy by removing superoxide anion, hydrogen peroxide, and peroxyl radical.

However, it is necessary to test agents and develop effective fertoprotective agents in the preservation of the ovarian reserve for OC patients.

FERTILITY PROSPECTS FOR HYSTERECTOMIZED WOMEN (BEYOND UTERUS TRANSPLANTATION)

Women who undergo hysterectomy need to consider other options such as surrogacy, even if they have cryopreserved oocytes. Successful uterus transplantation has been reported, but its application is still limited. High doses of immunosuppressive agents, the risk of cancer recurrence in immunocompromised patients, and the possible vascular abnormalities after pelvic radiation must be considered.

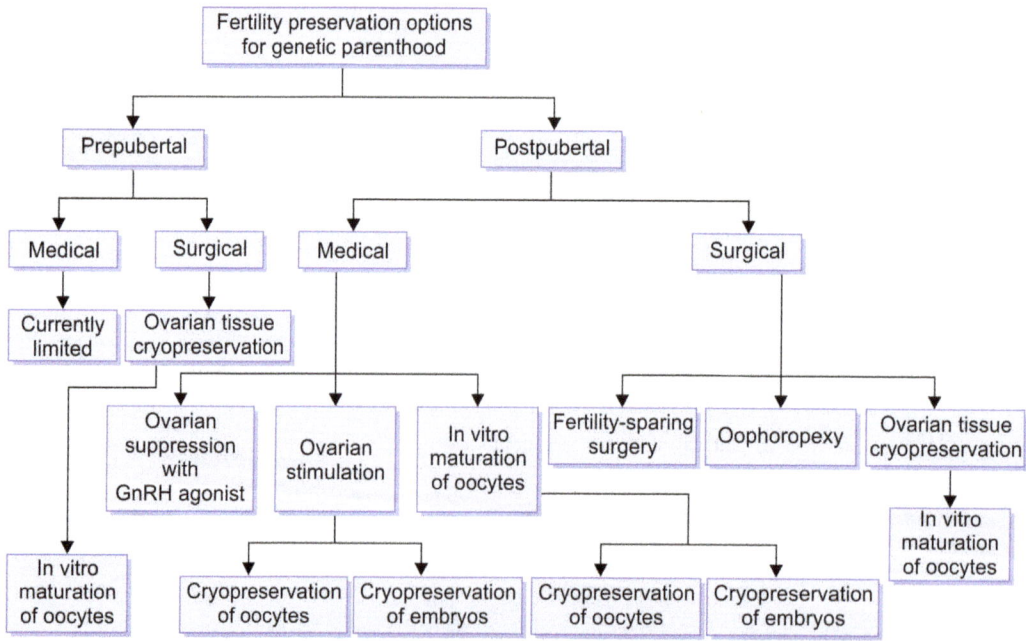

Flowchart 2: A simplified approach for fertility preservation in women of reproductive age.

(GnRH: gonadotropin-releasing hormone)

Source: Adapted from Pereira N, Schattman GL. Fertility preservation and sexual health after cancer therapy. J Oncol Pract. 2017;13:643-51.

However, it is emerging as a revolutionary approach even in gynecologic cancer patients with fertility preservation purposes.

CONCLUSION

The mean 5-year survival rate for OC is 47.4%, but it depends on the stage at the time of diagnosis.

The 5-year survival in:
- Stage I grade I->90%
- Stages IA and IB, stage II OC->70%
- Stage III about 39%
- Stage IV only 17%.

There is no scientific evidence to support a better prognosis with demolitive surgery and a conservative surgery can be proposed in the initial stages with adequate counseling. The choice must be based on an accurate staging and evaluation of prognostic factors such as grading and histotype. In case of negative prognostic factors, chemotherapy can have a fundamental role in allowing a fertility-sparing approach (**Flowchart 2**).

Unfortunately, there is no OC screening test except for an annual pelvic ultrasound. BRCA-mutated patients should undergo closer checks and monitoring of the markers.

Newer techniques such as uterus transplantation look promising, but are still far from common clinical practice. Till then, early diagnosis with fertility-sparing options are the only chance for these women to become pregnant. It carries significance especially in a resource-starved country like India where not being able to conceive is a social stigma as well.

The treating physician needs to be familiar with these options. They should be able to counsel the patients regarding the eligibility, indications, and limitations of fertility-sparing therapy.

CHAPTER 6

Uterine Fibroids in Adolescents

Priyanka Dilip Kumar

INTRODUCTION

The World Health Organization (WHO) identifies adolescents as young people between the ages of 10 years and 19 years and is often thought of as a healthy group but many serious diseases in adulthood have their roots in adolescence. Uterine fibroid, also referred to as uterine leiomyomata, uterine leiomyomas or uterine myomas is the most common benign tumor of the uterus occurring in women.[1] They are composed of smooth muscle layer accompanying connective tissues of the uterus. They exist sometimes singly but most often are multiple, or diffuse and if the uterus contains too many leiomyomata to count (**Fig. 1**), it is referred to as uterine leiomyomatosis.[2]

PREVALENCE

Uterine leiomyomas or fibroids are benign tumors originating from smooth muscle cells of the uterine wall. They are extremely common among women of reproductive age and it is estimated that about 60–80% of women may be affected at 50 years of age.[3] Unlike what occurs in adults, leiomyomas in adolescents are quite rare; only a few cases have been reported in the literature.[4] It is extremely rare in adolescence (<1%).[3]

The very word "fibroid" even though incidentally diagnosed during ultrasound examination will stir up a storm of anxieties, more so in a young girl who is just starting her reproductive life. It is an unlikely diagnosis in an adolescent but since the tumor depends on ovarian steroid hormones for its growth, ovarian activation at adolescence may trigger its growth in girls who are predisposed.[1]

SYMPTOMS

The clinical presentation of symptomatic uterine leiomyomas in adolescents may include:
- Heavy and prolonged menstrual bleeding
- Anemia (secondary to excessive menstrual blood loss)
- Pelvic pain and pressure
- Dysmenorrhea (painful menses)
- Urinary incontinence
- Constipation
- Lower back pain.

ETIOLOGY

The etiology of leiomyomas in adolescents and adults is generally unknown, but leiomyomas are known to grow in response to both estrogen and progesterone stimulation, and their prevalence increases throughout the reproductive years and is markedly reduced after menopause. Higher concentrations of estrogen and progesterone receptors, as well as aromatase, have been observed in fibroids compared to normal myometrial tissue (**Fig. 2**).[5] Studies have identified early age at menarche as a risk factor for the development of uterine leiomyomata, or fibroids.[6]

A genetic component of the pathogenesis of uterine fibroids has also been suggested. High-frequency mutations

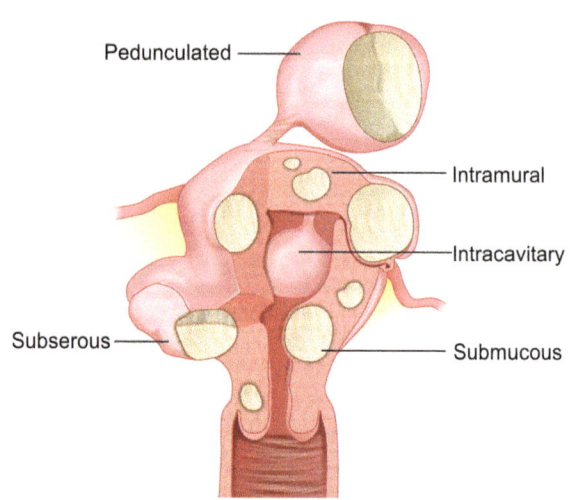

Fig. 1: Uterine leiomyomata.

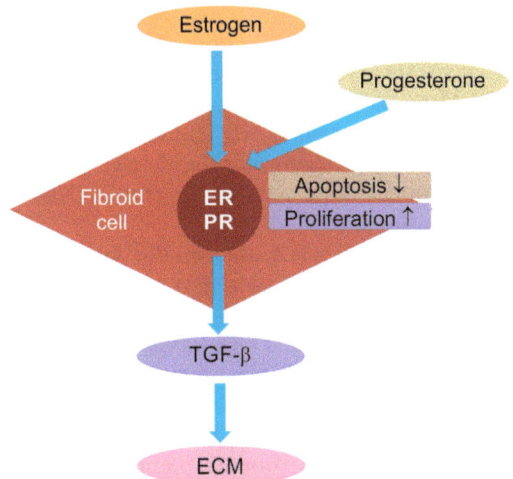

Fig. 2: Uterine fibroid pathophysiology.
(ECM: extracellular matrix; ER: estrogen receptor; PR: progesterone receptor; TGF-β: transforming growth factor-beta)

involving chromosomes 6, 7, 12, and 14 have been reported in uterine leiomyomas. It is not known, however, how these mutations initiate the cascade of events that eventually leads to the formation of a fibroid. Some theorists suggest that intrinsic myometrial anomalies and endometrial injury play important roles.[5]

SCREENING AND DIAGNOSIS

Uterine fibroids are rarely found in women under 20 years of age. When a pelvic mass in this age group is discovered, careful examination and radiographic imaging are imperative to arrive at the correct diagnosis.[7] The initial step in evaluating a woman with a pelvic mass is pelvic examination. If leiomyoma is suspected, the initial diagnostic adjunct should be ultrasonography, owing to its diagnostic accuracy, cost-effectiveness, and wide availability. Also, virginity-related issues may restrict the use of transvaginal ultrasound, magnetic resonance imaging provides precise identification and information about the numbers and location of these tumors. It also helps to differentiate uterine from adnexal masses, which are more prevalent at young age.[4] Computed tomography scanning is not recommended for the evaluation of uterine leiomyomas.[5]

TREATMENT OPTIONS

While there are universally accepted guidelines for treating uterine leiomyomas in adults that recommend minimally invasive surgical approaches, a management approach for this condition in the adolescent population is not well established. The treatment algorithm for uterine leiomyomas depends on the patient's age and family planning goals, as well as tumor size and symptomatology. Asymptomatic leiomyomas can be kept under observation, with regular evaluation to eliminate the possibility of malignant transformation.[5]

Surgical treatments such as myomectomy, myolysis, and hysterectomy can be employed when appropriate. Myomectomy is a common procedure performed for young women with symptomatic leiomyomas; it preserves fertility, does not interfere with the hormonal milieu of the developing adolescent, and is associated with a low recurrence rate. Myomectomy can be performed by laparotomy, laparoscopy, or hysteroscopy, depending on the number, size, and location of the fibroids.[5]

Medical treatments and minimally invasive procedures can be performed in some cases to allow a more rapid recovery. However, the use of such treatments in adolescents lacks supportive evidence and little is known about their applicability to this group.[5]

Uterine artery embolization (UAE) is an additional option. In this procedure, the ascending branches of the uterine artery supplying the leiomyomas are accessed and embolized to achieve complete loss of fibroid perfusion. This causes necrosis and shrinkage of the tumor. However, the potential complications associated with UAE (ovarian and Fallopian tube damage resulting from impaired blood flow) may limit its applicability in adolescents who desire to retain fertility.[5]

Medical management is only used for short-term therapy because of the significant risks associated with long-term treatment. Gonadotropin-releasing hormone agonists, selective estrogen receptor modulators antiprogestins (low-dose mifepristone), and aromatase inhibitors have all been utilized. There is limited evidence available regarding the efficacy of these medical interventions for managing uterine leiomyomas in the adolescent population.[5]

SUMMARY

- Uterine leiomyomas should be considered in adolescent women presenting with a pelvic mass and abdominal pain.
- Pelvic examination and ultrasonography are crucial to establish the diagnosis.
- Accurate evaluation of the etiology of these tumors is important for future counseling.
- The management of leiomyomas in this age group should be conservative, with the goal of preserving fertility.

- Myomectomy is the best procedure in the adolescent group, in view of preserving fertility.
- Physicians should offer pre- and postprocedure counseling regarding future fertility, recurrence following treatment, family planning options, and the importance of early and frequent antenatal visits when pregnant, as well as early completion of family size.

REFERENCES

1. Bassey D, Eduwem D, Inah G, Ekott M. Prevalence of uterine fibroid among adolescent school girls in Calabar Nigeria. IOSR J Dental Med Sci. 2016;15(3):74-5.
2. Nivethithai P, Nikhat SR, Rajesh BV. Uterine fibroids: a review. Indian J Pharm Pract. 2010;3(1):6-11.
3. Moroni RM, Vieira CS, Ferriani RA, Reis RM, Nogueira AA, Brito LG. Presentation and treatment of uterine leiomyoma in adolescence: a systematic review. BMC Womens Health. 2015;15:4.
4. Khodry MM, Abd-ellah AH, Tammam AA, Shazly SAM, Salem HT. Uterine leiomyomas in adolescents: a diagnostic and treatment dilemma—a case series. J Gynecol Surg. 2015;31(6):357-61.
5. Ernest A, Mwakalebela A, Mpondo BC. Uterine leiomyoma in a 19-year-old girl: case report and literature review. Malawi Med J. 2016;28(1):31-3.
6. Velez Edwards DR, Baird DD, Hartmann KE. Association of age at menarche with increasing number of fibroids in a cohort of women who underwent standardized ultrasound assessment. Am J Epidemiol. 2013;178(3):426-33.
7. Perkins JD, Hines RS, Prior DS. Uterine leiomyoma in an adolescent female. J Natl Med Assoc. 2009;101:611-3.

CHAPTER 7

Endometriosis in Adolescents

Sheela Mane

INTRODUCTION

Endometriosis is a gynecological condition defined as the presence of endometrial stroma and glands outside the normal uterus.[1] The inner menstruating layer of the uterus in women with endometriosis is termed the eutopic endometrium, whereas, the abnormal tissues outside the uterus are termed ectopic endometrium or "endometriotic lesions".[2] The disease often begins in adolescence, but is most often recognized after years of dysmenorrhea **(Fig. 1)**.[3]

Three types of endometriosis have been described—(1) peritoneal superficial endometriosis, (2) ovarian endometriomas, and (3) deep infiltrating endometriosis (DIE).[4]

PREVALENCE

The prevalence of endometriosis in adolescents undergoing laparoscopy for chronic pelvic pain is reported to be between 19 and 73%. Interestingly, endometriosis has also been identified in premenarcheal girls with some breast development.[1] The Endometriosis Association registry reports that 38% of women with endometriosis had symptoms starting before age 15 years and in such age group an average of 4.2 physician consultations are required before a diagnosis is reached, more than in any other age group.[5] A positive family history may be found more frequently in adolescents with endometriosis, a number of case series reporting a first degree relative with endometriosis in 25–30% of the patients.[6]

SYMPTOMS AND MARKERS IN ADOLESCENCE PREDICTING THE RISK OF ENDOMETRIOSIS

Initial delay in the diagnosis of endometriosis in adolescents may be because the pain is attributed to primary dysmenorrhea and hence considered a "normal" part of growing up. The presentation of endometriosis in adolescents often differs from that of adults. Contrary to the conventional cyclic pain associated with endometriosis, majority of adolescents diagnosed with endometriosis report both cyclic and acyclic pain. The pain is usually disruptive and affects their school, sports, and social activities.[5] Bowel and bladder symptoms are also common in adolescents. The localization in the ovary (ovarian endometrioma) is rare before 25 years.[3]

Symptoms and markers predicting the risk includes:
- Chronic pelvic pain, cyclic, and/or noncyclic
- Severe dysmenorrhea
- Noncontraceptive use of oral contraceptives for dysmenorrhea
- Dysmenorrhea resistant to nonsteroidal anti-inflammatory drugs (NSAIDs) and/or oral contraceptives
- Interference with daily living during menstruation, e.g. absenteeism from school
- Dyspareunia and/or pain on defecation during menstruation
- History of benign ovarian cysts
- Early age of menarche (≤12 years) (but not after 14 years)
- Family history of endometriosis.[7]

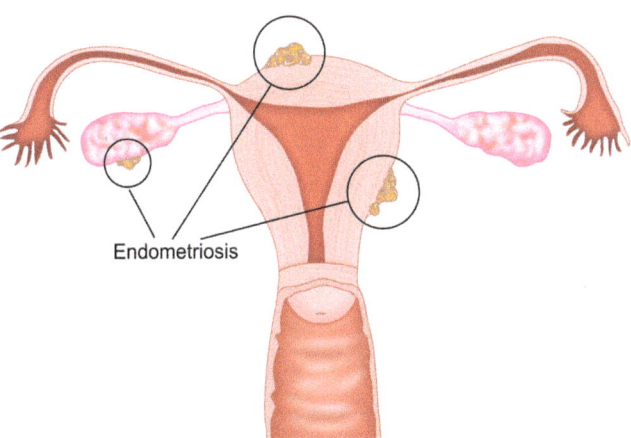

Fig. 1: Endometriosis.

PATHOPHYSIOLOGY

Several factors have been incriminated for endometriosis, while no single theory can explain the variety of symptoms. Like endometriosis in adults, endometriosis in adolescents is considered an inflammatory-mediated estrogen-dependent disorder. Estrogen produced by the ovaries, as well as estrogen produced locally by the endometriotic implants due to aromatase activity, promotes increased prostaglandin production, resulting in pain.[8] Obstructive anomalies of the female genital tract that enhances retrograde flow have been associated with endometriosis in the adolescent population. Other theories seeking to explain the origin of endometriosis have proposed that metaplastic cells transform into endometrial cells and endometrial cells metastasize through lymphatic and vascular channels, resulting in endometriosis. The most recent theories implicate an immune mechanism and suggest that a deficiency in cellular immunity allows the ectopic endometrial tissue to proliferate (**Fig. 2**).[9]

SCREENING AND DIAGNOSIS

The diagnosis is often delayed in the adolescent girls for a period of more than 6–8 years, if high index of suspicion is not there. A health risk screening tool such as the HEADSS assessment may assist the health care provider. HEADSS is a framework for history-taking that begins with topics the adolescent may have more comfort discussing and concludes with more sensitive questions: *H*ome or housing, *E*ducation and employment, *A*ctivities, *D*rugs, *S*exual activity and sexuality, and *S*uicide and depression. Privacy and confidentiality should be explained to both the adolescent and her family early on in the healthcare visit.

- Endometriosis has to be suspected in adolescents when they have severe dysmenorrhea, interfering with daily activities and school absenteeism not responding to NSAIDs when taken for pain relief.[10]
- Diagnosis in adolescents is through history, physical examination, risk factors, and family history combined with imaging technologies and biomarkers. A pelvic examination of the young adolescent may be limited; however, it is valuable to help rule out pelvic masses and obstructive outflow tract anomalies.[10]
- Inspection of the external genitalia, with separation and traction of the labia, may demonstrate low outflow tract anomalies.[5]
- A patent outflow can be determined by placing a Q-tip into the vaginal canal to assess its length and rule out transverse vaginal septum or vaginal agenesis.[5]
- Early onset progressive dysmenorrhea in adolescents should be investigated for the possibility of Müllerian anomaly with outflow tract obstruction.[10]
- Ultrasonography (USG) and magnetic resonance imaging (MRI) may be done. This may confirm diagnosis only in advanced lesions.[10]
- Measurement of CA-125 is nonspecific for diagnosing endometriosis and is generally not recommended.[5]
- Positive histology confirms the diagnosis, even though negative histology does not exclude it.[10]

PHENOTYPE OF ADOLESCENT VERSUS ADULT ENDOMETRIOSIS[11]

Phenotype of adolescent versus adult endometriosis is given in **Table 1**.

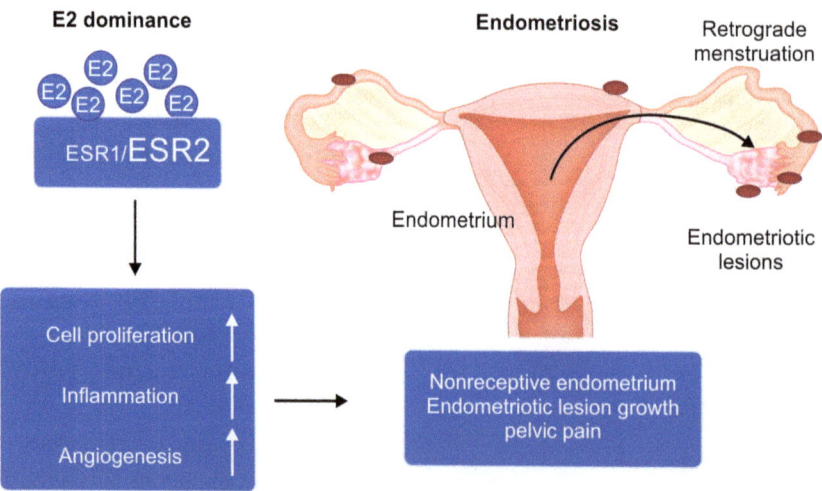

Fig. 2: Pathophysiology of endometriosis.

Table 1: Phenotype of adolescent versus adult endometriosis.

Adolescent endometriosis	Adult endometriosis
Symptoms: • Severe primary dysmenorrhea • Frequently resistant to oral contraceptive pill and nonsteroidal anti-inflammatory drugs	*Symptoms:* Moderate dysmenorrhea
Peritoneal: • Red, clear or vesicular implants • Minimal fibrosis	*Peritoneal:* • Black intraperitoneal implants • White, fibrotic
Ovarian endometrioma: • Cortex • Angiogenic adhesions • Stigma of inversion with implant • Invaginated cortex • Marble white • Thin angiogenic mucosal lining • Medulla • Stretched	*Ovarian endometrioma:* • Cortex • Dense adhesions • Stigma of inversion with implant • Invaginated cortex • Dark pigmented • Endometrial tufts • Thickened by fibrosis • Medulla • Smooth muscle metaplasia • Fibrosis and devascularization
Deep endometriosis: Seldom	*Deep endometriosis:* • Adenomyoma • Microendemetrioma
Concomitant pathology: Obstructive genital tract anomalies	*Concomitant pathology:* • Rectal and bladder endometriosis • Uterine adenomyosis

■ TREATMENT OPTIONS

The goals of treatment for adolescents with endometriosis are symptom control, prevention of further disease progression, and preservation of fertility. Medical and surgical options are available for the management of endometriosis. Most experts advocate prolonged medical therapy following laparoscopic diagnosis and excision of endometriosis.

Nonsteroidal Anti-inflammatory Drugs

Nonsteroidal anti-inflammatory drugs can be used as empiric treatment during management of dysmenorrhea in adolescents, even though the diagnosis of endometriosis has not been set yet.[1]

Combined Oral Contraceptives

Combined oral contraceptives (COCs) are typically the first-line treatment and can be used as well as empiric treatment. Acting by ovulation inhibition, they decrease gonadotropin levels and therefore reduce menstrual flow and cause decidualization of endometriotic implants. Another role of COCs is the decrease of cell proliferation, as well as the reduction of eutopic endometrium. According to Cochrane database of 2007, there are no sufficient data regarding long-term benefits of COC in the treatment of endometriosis.[1]

Progestins

Progesterone agents include medroxyprogesterone acetate (MPA) and 19-nortestosterone derivatives. These agents lead to decidualization and atrophy not only ectopic, but as well in eutopic endometrial tissue. It is important that up to 70–80% of girls suffering from endometriosis show symptoms improvement. On the other hand the benefits of long-term use of progestin therapy need to be weighed against impaired bone mineralization secondary to the hypoestrogenic environment induced by progestins, with the risk for osteoporotic fractures been yet unknown. Other side effects include weight gain, bloating, mood lability, and irregular bleeding.[1]

Newer progestins such as dienogest may help to relieve pain in adolescent girls and can be used for a longer period.[10] Dienogest is a fourth-generation progestin indicated as monotherapy at an oral dose of 2 mg once-daily in endometriosis. Dienogest is highly selective for the progesterone receptor, exhibiting strong progestational effects, and moderate antigonadotropic effects, with limited androgenic, glucocorticoid, or mineralocorticoid activity. Dienogest suppresses estradiol levels only moderately and, in a 6-month study in adults, did not alter mean lumbar spine bone mineral density (BMD). The safety and efficacy of dienogest for providing pain relief in the adult population have been confirmed in several clinical trials, differing in design, and ethnicity of populations.[12]

Gonadotropin-releasing Hormone Agonists

Gonadotropin-releasing hormone (GnRH) agonists are very effecting in treating adolescent endometriosis and alleviate symptoms associated with endometriosis. Acting by inducing menopause with binding to the GnRH receptors in the pituitary, they result to cessation of pituitary gonadotropin release and subsequently to amenorrhea. It is of great importance to remember that the use of GnRH agonists alone is generally limited to patients more than 16 years of age and for a period no more than 6 months.[1]

Danazol

Danazol is a 17-ethinyl testosterone derivative with an efficacy being equivalent to a variety of GnRH agonists in treating endometriosis. Its androgenic effects, affecting sex-hormone-binding globulin levels, resulting in an increase of free testosterone. It causes androgenic side effects (weight gain, acne, irreversible deepening of the voice, etc.). Due to the fact that this agent is poorly tolerated by adolescents is not widely utilized in endometriosis management.[1]

Surgical Treatment

Laparoscopy is preferred over laparotomy in adolescents. The laparoscopic procedure should be both diagnostic and therapeutic and to be preferably done by a senior consultant with experience in treating endometriosis. Endometriotic implants have variable morphology, which has been described in the revised American Society of Reproductive Medicine (ASRM) classification of endometriosis **(Figs. 3A to H)**.[9] Surgery should be timed in the follicular phase of menstrual cycle. This will help minimize recurrences and adhesions. First port should be intraumbilical and the lateral ports should be placed close to the pubic bone for cosmetic superiority. Surgery has been shown to be effective in improving endometriosis symptoms; reported improvement rates range from 38 to 100%. Various techniques are used, including laser vaporization, unipolar or bipolar coagulation, and endocoagulation; no one technique has been shown to be superior to any other. However, symptoms generally return in the majority of patients after 1 year without further treatment and so surgery alone is not considered adequate treatment in the adolescent patient population. These patients need to be put on long-term suppressive medical therapy as described earlier.

The American College of Obstetricians and Gynecologists has put forth a stepwise treatment algorithm **(Flowchart 1)** for the care of adolescents presenting with dysmenorrhea.[5]

Follow-up

Since endometriosis can be a life-long disease, careful follow-up of the adolescents after surgical diagnosis and treatment is important. The findings should be clearly explained to the patient and her caretakers. Patient should be reviewed every 3–6 months. During this time, her symptoms should be monitored closely and the girl should be educated about the possible, long-term nature of endometriosis and the need to minimize the number of pelvic surgeries. Concerns about fertility and quality of life should be addressed. Unless contraindicated, most patients should be put on OCP after surgery. If the patient does not respond to surgery or has recurrence of symptoms, other modes of long-term, medical therapy are considered and an investigation into other causes of pelvic pain is warranted. Gastroenterology, psychology, and urology experts should be consulted if required and this ensures appropriate evaluation of such patients for coexisting diseases and optimizes their care.

■ SUMMARY

- Endometriosis is a progressive disease and a significant number of women with endometriosis report symptoms starting in adolescence.
- Pain is the main symptom, especially dysmenorrhea and chronic pelvic pain.
- The diagnosis is often delayed, leading to suffering for several years and, for this reason, there is a need to early diagnosis of endometriosis.
- Primary goals are alleviation of pain symptoms, avoidance of disease recurrence, and assurance of future fertility preservation.
- Nonsteroidal anti-inflammatory drugs and COCs can be used as first-line medical treatment during management of adolescent endometriosis.
- Dienogest is a fourth-generation progestin which has shown promising results in adolescent endometriosis with improved safety compared to conventional progestins.
- Laparoscopy (with biopsy) is the only way to diagnose endometriosis in the adolescent population, and surgical management has been shown to be beneficial in reducing pain, infertility, and progression or recurrence of disease.
- Postoperative hormonal suppression helps reduce pain symptoms and recurrence of endometriomas.

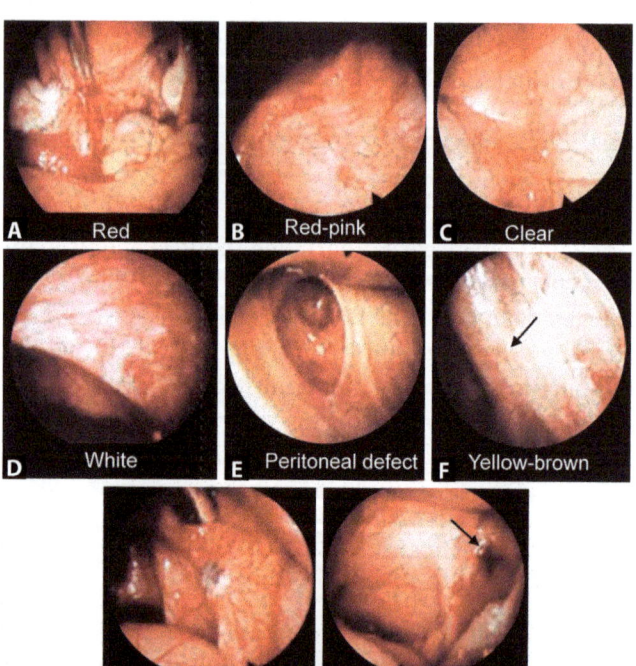

Figs. 3A to H: Classification of endometriosis.

Flowchart 1: Stepwise treatment algorithm for the care of adolescents.

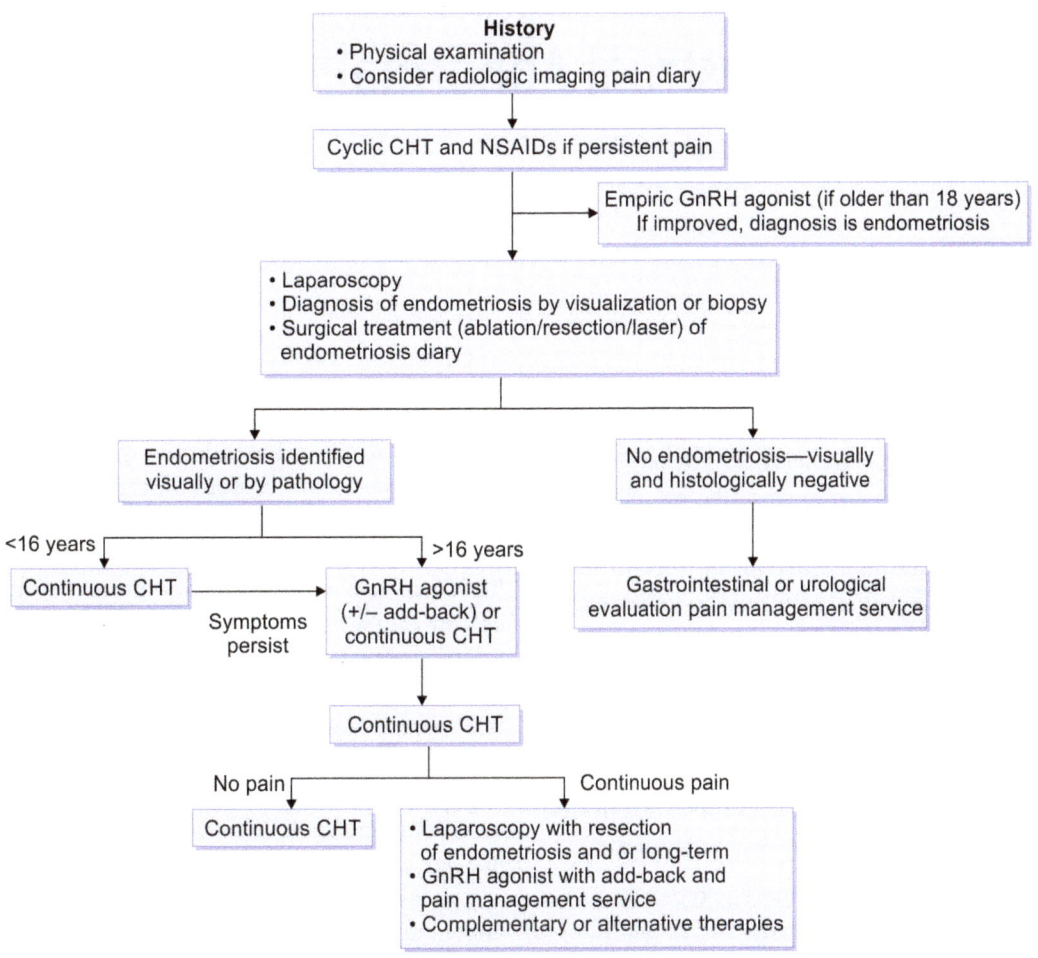

(CHT: cyclic hormone thermotherapy; NSAID; nonsteroidal anti-inflammatory drug; GnRH: gonadotropin-releasing hormone)

REFERENCES

1. Deligeoroglou E, Karountzos V, Tsimaris P, Ekott M. Endometriosis in adolescence: challenges and opportunities for managing future infertility. Int J Gynecol Clin Pract. 2018;5:145.
2. Nguyen AT, Markham R, Manconi F. Endometriosis in the Adolescents. Gynaecol Perinatol. 2018;2(1):181-91.
3. Dessole M, Melis GB, Angioni S. Endometriosis in adolescence. Obstetr Gynecol Int. 2012;869191:4.
4. Cirstoiu M, Bodean O, Secara D, Munteanu O, Cirstoiu C. Case study of a rare form of endometriosis. J Med Life. 2013;6(1):68-71.
5. Nanthakumar MP, Arumugam SC. Adolescent endometriosis. Int J Reprod Contracept Obstet Gynecol. 2017;6(8):3213-8.
6. Sarıdoğan E. Adolescent endometriosis. Eur J Obstet Gynecol Reprod Biol. 2017;209:46-9.
7. Tanbo TG, Qvigstad E. Endometriosis in adolescence: predictive markers and management. Acta Obstet Gynecol Scand. 2013;92:491-5.
8. American College of Obstetricians and Gynecologists. Dysmenorrhea and endometriosis in the adolescent. ACOG Committee Opinion No. 760. Obstet Gynecol. 2018;132:e249-58.
9. Laufer MR, Sanfilippo J, Rose G. Adolescent endometriosis: diagnosis and treatment approaches. J Pediatr Adolesc Gynecol. 2003;16(3 Suppl):S3-11.
10. FOGSI Endometriosis Committee. (2014-2016) Good Clinical Practice Recommendations on Endometriosis. [online] Available from: https://www.fogsi.org/wp-content/uploads/2017/01/GCRP-2017-final.pdf [Last accessed January, 2020].
11. Benagiano G, Guo SW, Puttemans P, Gordts S, Brosens I, Brosens I. Progress in the diagnosis and management of adolescent endometriosis: an opinion. Reprod Biomed Online. 2018;36(1):102-14.
12. Ebert AD, Dong L, Merz M, Kirsch B, Francuski M, Böttcher B. Dienogest 2 mg daily in the treatment of adolescents with clinically suspected endometriosis: The VISanne Study to Assess Safety in ADOlescents. J Pediatr Adolesc Gynecol. 2017;30(5):560-7.

CHAPTER 8

Menstrual Abnormalities in Adolescents

Jitendra Mane, Parag Biniwale

■ INTRODUCTION

Transition from childhood to adolescence is brought about by multiple events which are played like an orchestra. Appearance of secondary sexual characters and accelerated growth followed by menarche are an important event during adolescence which marks the onset of reproductive capabilities and completion of puberty. As per the World Health Organization (WHO), adolescence age is between 10 and 19 years. Although median age at menarche has remained relatively stable between 12 and 13 years,[1,2] but environmental factors, including socioeconomic conditions, nutrition, and access to preventive health care, may influence the timing and progression of puberty.

Normal and abnormal menses: Menarche typically occurs within 2–3 years after thelarche (breast budding at Tanner stage IV breast development). By age 15 years, 98% of females will have had menarche. An evaluation for primary amenorrhea should be considered for any adolescent who has not reached menarche by age 15 years or has not done so within 3 years of thelarche. Menstrual abnormalities are common during adolescence due to slow maturation of the hypothalamic-pituitary-ovarian (HPO) axis and can last 2–5 years after menarche. Most girls bleed for 2–7 days during their first menses with 90% of cycles within the range of 21–45 days, although short cycles of less than 20 days and long cycles of more than 45 days may occur. By the third year after menarche, 60–80% of menstrual cycles are 21–34 days long, as is typical of adults.[3,4]

■ ETIOLOGY

Heavy menstrual bleeding (HMB) is defined as excessive menstrual blood loss that interferes with a woman's physical, social, emotional, or material quality of life. A number of medical conditions can cause abnormal uterine (AUB) bleeding characterized by unpredictable timing and variable amount of flow. Although a long interval between cycles is common in adolescence due to anovulation, it is statistically uncommon for girls and adolescents to remain amenorrheic for more than 3 months or 90 days. Girls and adolescents with more than 3 months between periods should be evaluated. Bleeding once identified as abnormal may be categorized as per cause in the acronym PALM-COEIN—Polyp, Adenomyosis, Leiomyoma, Malignancy as structural causes and Coagulopathy, Ovulatory dysfunction, Endometrial, Iatrogenic, Not otherwise classified as nonstructural causes.[5] This helps to plan management of patient. AUB caused due to anovulation followed by coagulation defects is more frequent in adolescence. Androgen excess conditions like polycystic ovary syndrome (PCOS), congenital adrenal hyperplasia, and androgen producing tumors which cause anovulatory bleeding may be suggested by the presence of obesity, hirsutism, and acne. Hypothalamic dysfunction may be indicated by eating disorders, stress, and excess physical activity. Hypothyroidism and hyperprolactinemia are common endocrine causes of anovulation. 20% of adolescence girls have bleeding deficits who present with AUB. von Willebrand disease, platelet function defects, thrombocytopenia, clotting factor deficiencies, and immune thrombocytopenic purpura or thrombotic thrombocytopenic purpura can present with HMB.[6] Common medications including hormonal contraceptive pills, anticoagulants, and selective serotonin reuptake inhibitors may cause alterations in menstrual bleeding. Structural causes of HMB such as polyps, leiomyoma, or vascular malformations occur rarely in adolescents, but may be considered in those who are refractory to treatment as anticipated. Pregnancy and sexually transmitted infection (STI) should always be kept in back of the mind.

■ CLINICAL PRESENTATIONS

When adolescent girl presents to outpatient department (OPD) or casualty with complaints of AUB, detailed history taking is very important. Detailed question about her menstrual history including the age of menarche and the menstrual frequency, regularity, duration, and volume of flow.

As per the American College of Obstetricians and Gynecologists (ACOG) Committee opinion 651 December 2015,[7] menstrual abnormalities that may require evaluation are:

- If *no menarche*: (a) After 3 years of thelarche, (b) 14 years of age along with signs of hirsutism or history of dietary disorder or excessive physical activity, and (c) By 15 years of age.
- If frequency of cycles: (a) Every 21 days or less, (b) 45 days and more, and (c) 90 days apart even for one cycle.
- If duration and amount of flow: (a) More than 7 days and (b) soaks more than one pad or tampon every 1–2 hours.
- History of bruising, recurrent epistaxis or gum bleeding, surgery-associated excessive bleeding, and family history of a bleeding disorder.

Quantifying blood loss may be difficult as the adolescent may not be aware of normal and excess flow. Pictorial menstrual assessment can be done to ascertain blood loss. The presence of cramping and/or clots and number of pads/tampons soaked can be useful information to assess amount of bleeding. Anemia which is a result of HMB in adolescents can lead to symptoms like fatigue, headache, and decreased cognition specifically affecting verbal learning and memory that suggest significant and prolong bleeding.

Psychologically girls may suffer from depressed mood or anxiety due to heavy bleeding for which she may skip school, avoid participating in games, and outdoor activities.

Approximately 50% of adolescent girls with bleeding disorder present with heavy menstrual bleeding. At menarche, rest may not present until cycles become ovulatory.[8] Gynecological presentation of bleeding disorder would be recurrent hemorrhagic corpus luteum with or without rupture.

Sexual history is a must to rule out pregnancy-associated complications and risk of STIs. Eliciting drug history of contraceptive pills usage and anticoagulants is also important. Other symptoms for evaluation of systemic disorders must be taken.

PHYSICAL EVALUATION

Detailed physical examination of the patient who presents with HMB should be carried out which in most cases will be normal. However, hemodynamic instability may be present where rapid interventions are needed. Signs of anemia and bleeding disorders in form of pallor, bruises, and petechiae may be present. Obesity, acne, hirsutism, and acanthosis nigricans if present suggest PCOS. Appropriateness of sexual maturity level should be assessed if not then local trauma also needs to be considered. An abdominal examination should be done to assess for any palpable pelvic mass which should be further evaluated. In adolescent girls with HMB, speculum examination typically is not required. However, vaginal examination is possible in a girl who is sexually active.

INVESTIGATIONS

Adolescents presenting with AUB must be evaluated with complete blood count with white blood cell differential and platelet count. Blood group should be done if need for transfusion arises. Serum ferritin levels need to be checked for iron stores.[9] Further evaluation should be guided by the history and examination findings. Screening for bleeding disorder should be done particularly for von Willebrand disease with activated partial thromboplastin time (aPTT), von Willebrand antigen, von Willebrand activity, von Willebrand factor: ristocetin cofactor (vWF:RCo), and factor VIII levels.

If patient is on estrogen, it will show normal values of vWF levels hence it is advised to stop estrogen for few weeks and repeat the test. Sexually active adolescents should be tested for pregnancy and STIs including gonorrhea and *Chlamydia*. Hormonal test for thyroid function and prolactin levels must be offered. In those with signs of PCOS or insulin resistance, laboratory testing should be offered accordingly.

Imaging in the form of transabdominal ultrasonography which is more appropriate than transvaginal should be obtained in patients with features of PCOS, or those not responsive to initial medical management, or with pelvic mass or suspecting pregnancy-related complications.[10]

MANAGEMENT

Abnormal uterine bleeding during adolescent period is usually due to anovulation which is self-limited and resolves once the HPO axis matures for which reassurance and supportive care are given. Most of the girls present in OPD with AUB are managed as outpatient. However, some may present as emergency with HMB for whom energetic management is warranted to reduce morbidity **(Flowchart 1)**.

Aim of management of acute bleeding is to control present episode of acute bleeding and to have reduced menstrual blood loss during subsequent periods which is achieved by medical management. Surgical options are

Flowchart 1: Approaches to testing and management.

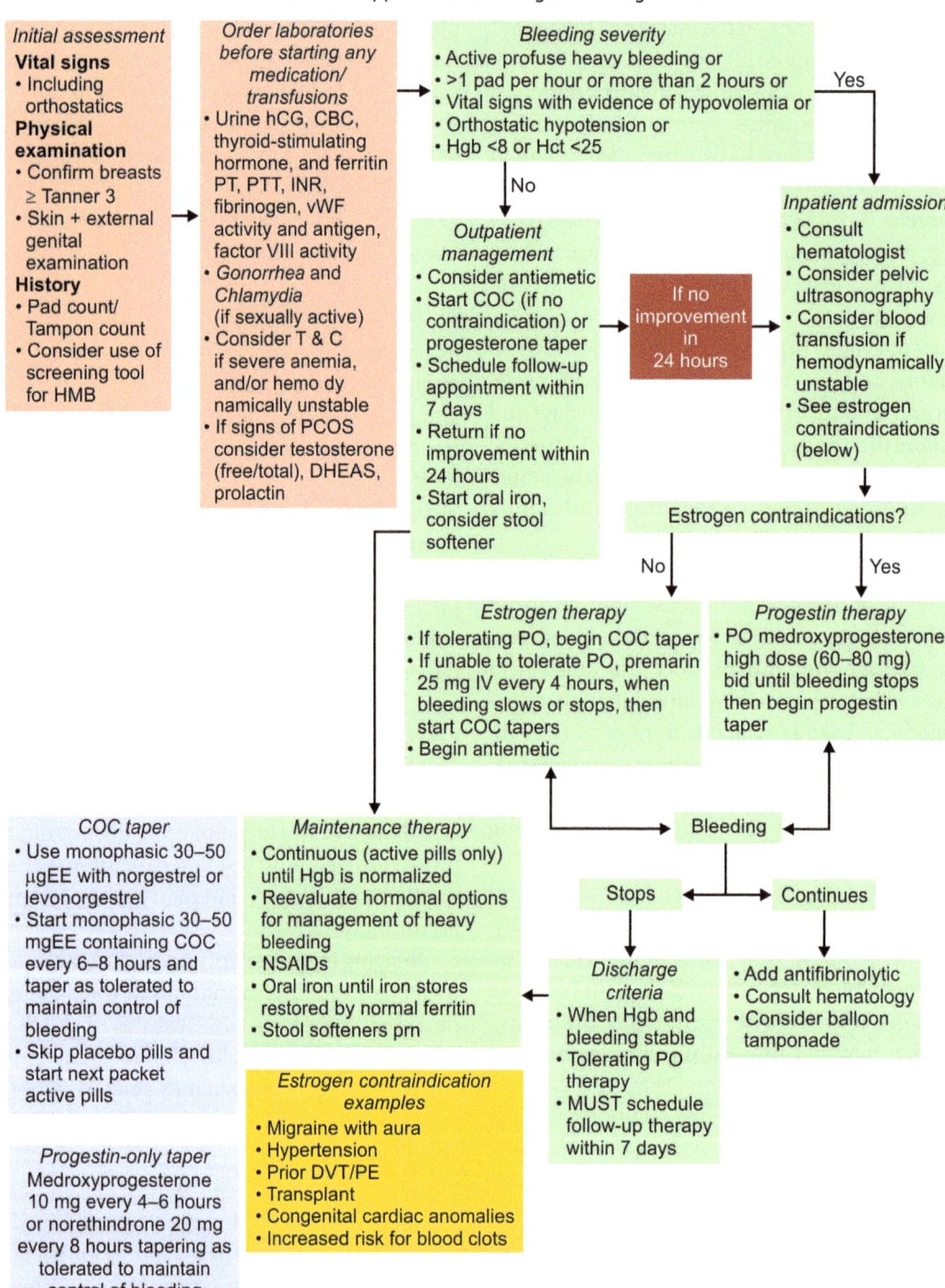

(bid: two times a day; CBC: complete blood count; COC: combined oral contraceptive; DHEAS: dehydroepiandrosterone sulfate; DVT: deep vein thrombosis; EE: ethinyl estradiol; hCG: human chorionic gonadotropin; Hct: hematocrit; Hgb: hemoglobin; HMB: heavy menstrual bleeding; INR: international normalized ratio; IV: intravenously; NSAIDs: nonsteroidal anti-inflammatory drugs; PCOS: polycystic ovary syndrome; PE: pulmonary embolism; PO: per oral; prn: as needed; PT: prothrombin time; PTT: partial thromboplastin time; T & C: type and cross; vWF: von Willebrand factor)
Source: Adapted from Ely JW, Kennedy CM, Clark EC, et al. Abnormal uterine bleeding: a management algorithm. J Am Board Fam Med. 2006;19:590-602.

utilized when medical management fails. Depending on hemodynamic status, resuscitative measures are initiated along with hormonal therapy and iron replacement.

Nonhormonal Therapy

Antifibrinolytics

Tranexamic acid in oral (1.3 g thrice a day) and intravenous (10 mg/kg maximum 600 mg/dose thrice a day) form is used as first-line drug as it reduces 40–50% blood loss. The action is by reversibly blocking lysine sites on plasminogen thus inhibits fibrinolysis. In view of both tranexamic acid and combined oral contraceptives (COCs) having thrombotic tendencies, there use together is of concern[11] however the available limited literature has not identified an increased risk of venous thromboembolism[12] when used after failure of monotherapy, i.e., estrogen alone or tranexamic acid alone.

Prostaglandin Synthesis Inhibitors

Mefenamic acid 500 mg thrice a day for 7 days is the most commonly used molecule for reducing menstrual blood loss and pain due to its different mechanism of action of inhibiting prostaglandin synthases enzyme as well as binding and inhibiting the prostaglandin receptors which leads to improve endometrial hemostasis. This help in reducing 25–40% blood loss.

Hormonal Medical Therapy

By menarche, most girls have completed 95% of their growth with epiphyseal plate closure so treatment with estrogen should not be much concern for the treatment of HMB. If no contraindications, estrogen is used in treating acute HMB by monophasic combined oral contraceptive pills (OCPs) (COCs) (in 30–50 µg ethinyl estradiol formulation) that can be used every 6–8 hours until cessation of bleeding. The high doses of estrogen induce nausea and vomiting for which antiemetics should be added.

If bleeding stops typically within 24–48 hours, a combined OCP tapering regimen should be initiated, i.e., taper to three times daily for 3 days and then to twice daily to complete a 21-day course of pills. Then the patient starts a new pack of COC without using the placebo pills. If bleeding does not stop or does not improve significantly within 24–48 hours, then hematologist consultation should be sought. COCs should be continued in minimal doses at which no breakthrough bleeding takes place till such time the general condition of patient improves and adequate rise in hemoglobin. Typically, a three cycle therapy is used for regularization of menstrual cycle.

If estrogen is contraindicated or not well-tolerated orally, then medroxyprogesterone acetate (MPA) 10–20 mg every 6–12 hours or norethisterone acetate 5–10 mg every 6 hours for 7 days should taper the dose. Depot preparation of MPA is not suitable for acute HMB treatment due to the difficulty in titrating dose-related effect or to discontinue if there are adverse effects.

Other Supportive Care

Need for blood transfusion in adolescence AUB is only in exceptional situations like hemodynamically unstable patient or those with severe symptoms of anemia (e.g., tachycardia, lethargy, syncope, and tachypnea). Recommendations are for restrictive transfusion practice to patients with hemoglobin less than 7 g/dL.[13] These otherwise healthy adolescents tolerate hemoglobin levels less than 7 g/dL and a decision to transfuse should be based on hemodynamic status. Iron should be started concurrently with hormonal therapy.

Nonpharmacological Management

Nonmedical procedures should be considered when there is a lack of response to medical therapy in patients who are clinically unstable despite initial measures or when severe heavy bleeding warrants further investigation such as an examination under anesthesia. Suction curettage and intrauterine balloon can be considered. However, different invasive options are considered in this group of patients only in life-threatening scenario as they affect future fertility.

Intrauterine Balloon

This intervention is easily available, effective which can help avoid invasive procedures. Foley catheter is inserted easily through the cervix and balloon inflated with saline until resistance of the myometrium is felt. The catheter kept in place for 12–24 hours while other medical therapies are being administered, then gradually balloon is deflated or the balloon can be removed after 24 hours with observation for bleeding. An advantage of the balloon is the ability to simultaneously monitor for uterine bleeding. A risk associated with this procedure is infection which can be reduced by using antibiotics while balloon is in place. Other risks are uterine perforation and endometrial lining damage.[14,15]

Uterine Evacuation

Suction evacuation may be done if ultrasonography is suggestive of intrauterine clot or decidual cast or pregnancy completions. Sharp curettage should be avoided as this can lead to excessive bleeding in patients with bleeding disorder. In selected patients, therapeutic dilation and curettage remove fragile endometrium, thereby helping in hemostasis by restoring synchronized proliferation of endometrium.[16] Hysteroscopy may be performed if intrauterine pathology is suspected or if a tissue sampling is desired.

Maintenance Therapy

After correction of acute HMB, maintenance hormonal therapy can include combined hormonal contraceptives, oral and injectable progestins, and levonorgestrel-releasing intrauterine devices (LNG-IUDs). Nonhormonal treatment for anemia includes oral iron supplementation and dietary optimization. COCs, the transdermal contraceptive patch, the vaginal contraceptive ring, and the LNG-IUD all have been shown to reduce menstrual blood loss. COCs, monophasic pills that contain 30–50 μg of ethinyl estradiol with a second-generation progesterone, should be chosen as first-line therapy as they stabilize the endometrium better then low-dose preparations. COCs with 50 μg ethinyl estradiol may be used if breakthrough bleeds. Progestin therapy is another option for adolescents and women who cannot tolerate estrogen-containing therapy or in whom estrogen is contraindicated. Progesterone-only contraceptive pill can be used, but it has short half-life that can lead to breakthrough bleeding and decreased contraceptive efficacy in adolescents. Norethisterone 5 mg titrated in doses of 5–15 mg daily is used for menstrual suppression. Depot MPA 150 mg injections can be used, but there is increased risk of intramuscular hematoma formation. LNG-IUD can be better choice for adolescent as daily medication may pose difficulty. LNG-IUD has demonstrated reduced blood loss in HMB, but its efficacy in bleeding disorder is not well-established.[17,18] Also there are concerns of increased bleeding while insertion of device. However, in setting of nulligravida adolescent, LNG-IUD should be used after due counseling. In these cases of HMB, patients should be counseled about the higher risk of expulsion rates. As iron deficiency anemia is more prevalent in adolescents with AUB, treatment with oral or parenteral iron is recommended. Oral iron in the dosage of 60–120 mg/day needs to be prescribed for 3–6 months depending on severity of anemia.[19,20]

Abnormal uterine bleeding in adolescence is common, but may significantly impair quality of life. Although it is often due to HPO axis immaturity, but it may be an important sentinel for underlying bleeding disorder and needs multidisciplinary management approach. Medical treatment modalities available are effective solemnly surgical options resorted. These girls may require long duration of hormonal and iron therapy for management of HMB and anemia.

CONCLUSION

Menstrual abnormality is the common presentation for which adolescents sought medical attention. Even though anovulatory cycles are the most common etiology, sinister bleeding disorders need to be kept in mind. Multidisciplinary approach is required for evaluation and management of adolescents with HMB. Medical management is the-first line of management with HMB, surgical approach is needed only in few if medical means fail. Antifibrinolytics and hormonal medical therapy is the mainstay of medical approach for control and long-term management of AUB. Correction of anemia with long- term iron therapy need not be over emphasized for overall well-being of adolescents.

REFERENCES

1. Chumlea WC, Schubert CM, Roche AF, Kulin HE, Lee PA, Himes JH, et al. Age at menarche and racial comparisons in US girls. Pediatrics. 2003;111:110-3.
2. Finer LB, Philbin JM. Trends in ages at key reproductive transitions in the United States, 1951–2010. Womens Health Issues. 2014;24:e271-9.
3. Widholm O, Kantero RL. A statistical analysis of the menstrual patterns of 8,000 Finnish girls and their mothers. Acta Obstet Gynecol Scand Suppl. 1971;14:Suppl 14:1-36.
4. Hickey M, Balen A. Menstrual disorders in adolescence: investigation and management. Hum Reprod Update. 2003;9:493-504.
5. American College of Obstetricians and Gynecologists. ACOG Committee opinion no. 557: Management of acute abnormal uterine bleeding in nonpregnant reproductive-aged women. Obstet Gynecol. 2013;121:891-6.
6. Committee on Adolescent Health Care; Committee on Gynecologic Practice. Committee Opinion No. 580: von Willebrand disease in women. Obstet Gynecol. 2013;122:1368-73.
7. ACOG Committee Opinion No. 651: Menstruation in Girls and Adolescents: Using the Menstrual Cycle as a Vital Sign. Obstet Gynecol. 2015;126:e143-6.
8. Dowlut-McElroy T, Williams KB, Carpenter SL, Strickland JL. Menstrual patterns and treatment of heavy menstrual bleeding in adolescents with bleeding disorders. J Pediatr Adolesc Gynecol. 2015;28:499-501.
9. Johnson S, Lang A, Sturm M, O'Brien SH. Iron deficiency without anaemia: a common yet under-recognized

diagnosis in young women with heavy menstrual bleeding. J Pediatr Adolesc Gynecol. 2016;29:628-31.
10. Pecchioli Y, Oyewumi L, Allen LM, Kives S. The utility of routine ultrasound in the diagnosis and management of adolescents with abnormal uterine bleeding. J Pediatr Adolesc Gynecol. 2017;30:239-42.
11. Lexicomp. (2019). Facts and Comparisons. [online] Available from: http://fco.factsandcomparisons.com/lco/action/home. [Last accessed April, 2020].
12. Thorne JG, James PD, Reid RL. Heavy menstrual bleeding: is tranexamic acid a safe adjunct to combined hormonal contraception [commentary]? Contraception. 2018;98:1-3.
13. Napolitano LM, Kurek S, Luchette FA, Anderson GL, Bard MR, Bromberg W, et al. Clinical practice guideline: red blood cell transfusion in adult trauma and critical care. Crit Care Med. 2009;37:3124-57.
14. James AH, Kouides PA, Abdul-Kadir R, Dietrich JE, Edlund M, Federici AB. Evaluation and management of acute menorrhagia in women with and without underlying bleeding disorders: consensus from an international expert panel. Eur J Obstet Gynecol Reprod Biol. 2011;158:124-34.
15. Hamani Y, Ben-Shachar I, Kalish Y, Porat S. Intrauterine balloon tamponade as a treatment for immune thrombocytopenic purpura-induced severe uterine bleeding. Fertil Steril. 2010;94:2769.e13-5.
16. Handa VL, Le LV. Te Linde's Atlas of Gynecologic Surgery, 12th edition. Philadelphia: Wolters Kluwer; 2019.
17. Health Quality Ontario. Levonorgestrel-releasing intrauterine system (52 mg) for idiopathic heavy menstrual bleeding: a health technology assessment. Ont Health Technol Assess Ser. 2016;16:1-119.
18. Irvine GA, Campbell-Brown MB, Lumsden MA, Heikkilä A, Walker JJ, Cameron IT. Randomised comparative trial of the levonorgestrel intrauterine system and norethisterone for treatment of idiopathic menorrhagia. Br J Obstet Gynaecol. 1998;105:592-8.
19. Centers for Disease Control and Prevention. Recommendations to prevent and control iron deficiency in the United States. MMWR Recomm Rep. 1998;47:1-29.
20. American College of Obstetricians and Gynecologists. ACOG Practice Bulletin No. 95: anemia in pregnancy. Obstet Gynecol. 2008;112:201-7.

CHAPTER 9

Teenage Pregnancies and Abortions: Today's Scenario

Munjal Jayeshkumar Pandya, Janki Pandya

■ INTRODUCTION

Teenage pregnancy is considered as pregnancy in females of age between 10 and 19 years of age, often described as adolescent pregnancy. Teenage pregnancy is on rise since last few decades. Changing generation, with easy access to all the knowledge on internet and without proper maturity and thought process, has contributed a lot in recent times. There has been a huge generation gap between generation of parents who thought sex education as a taboo, and the generation of teenagers of recent times, for many of whom, it is perceived as signs of modernization and fun. Westernization, without inculcating values along with following societal imperfect role models has costed hugely. Conceiving in teenage years has grave implications on conceptus, the mother as well as the family. Many of these pregnancies end up in induced abortions.

■ GLOBAL PERSPECTIVE

Around 16 million girls between age group of 15 and 19 years give birth every year in developing nations.[1] Globally, adolescent birth rate has fallen from 65 births per 1,000 women in 1990 to 47 births per 1,000 women in 2015.[2] Globally, around 90% of these adolescent births happen within marriage.[1,3]

Developing versus Developed

Approximately 95% of total teenage births occur in low and middle-income countries.[4] Low-income countries show five times higher births of adolescent pregnancies as compared to high-income countries, while middle-income countries have around twice the rate as compared to high-income countries. Globally, there are many countries, like Caribbean, sub-Saharan Africa, and Latin America, which have higher rates of teenage pregnancies outside marriage as compared to Asian countries. Most of countries of sub-Saharan Africa were found to have approximately 70% of adolescent women sexually active, and more than 50% of total births were noted amongst adolescent women.[5]

Globally, in poorest regions, 1 in 3 adolescent females become pregnant. India, Bangladesh, Brazil, Congo, Nigeria, Ethiopia, and United States are those seven countries, which constitute half of the adolescent pregnancies all over the world.[5]

Netherlands has the lowest teenage pregnancy rates amongst developed countries, while England and Wales showed teenage pregnancy rates of around 45/1,000. Japan, Sweden, Norway, and Finland showed lower rates, while Iceland and New Zealand showed higher rates.[6]

USA showed the highest teenage pregnancy rate amongst developed countries, with approximately 1 in every 11 girls aged 15–19 years getting pregnant each year. According to 1998 data, birth rate in 15–19 years girls was 51.1 live births/1,000.[7] Gradually, the rate dropped down to 34.3/1,000 in age group of 15–19 years in 2010.[8] USA faced sharp rise in teenage pregnancies in mid 1970s, which lead to legalization of abortion and development and promotion of various methods of contraception, helping the downward fall in the trend.[9]

Indian Scenario

India legalized abortion in form of medical termination of Pregnancy Act of 1971, after steep rise in illegal abortions in 1960s and 1970s, resulting in decline in maternal morbidity and mortality. At the start of 1990s, rates of illegal abortions were very high with ratio of illegal to legal abortion 11:1, with rise in maternal morbidity and mortality.[10] India was the country with highest number of abortions all over the world in various studies. According to one study, around 9 million abortions occurred in India in 1995.[11]

India, as a developing nation, has been facing a lot of challenges due to population growth, with teenagers comprising of around 26% of total population.[12] According to

World Health Organization (WHO), approximately, 26% of females get married by the age of 15 years, and around 54% of females get married by the age of 18 years in India.[13] Census 2001 concluded that approximately 20% of 1.5 million females under age of 15 years, were found to be pregnant. According to NFHS-4 (National Family Health Survey) published in 2015-2016, approximately 11.9% girls (14.1% in rural area and 6.9% in urban area) got married in the age group of 15-19 years. Out of all the states, the worst were Bihar (42.5%), West Bengal (41.6%), and Jharkhand (37.9%). Amongst age group of 15-19 years, 30.8% of illiterate females got married, while the rate of child marriage was only 2.4% in 15-19 years of age group with higher education. 31.5% of married females between ages of 15 and 19 years had their first child. Almost 25% of "first" babies were born in the age group of 15-16 years, while another 26-27% had it by the age of 17 years. Around 31% had their first child by the age of 18 years.[14]

Abortion

As most of these pregnancies are unwanted and unplanned, around 30-60% of these end up in abortions. Around 23 million girls between ages 15 and 19 years in developing nations do not have access/knowledge of contraception. Around 3.9 million girls between 15 and 19 years of age undergo unsafe abortions globally, every year.[15] Many a times, the fear of nonacceptance by society and immaturity leads to illegal-septic abortions, costing hugely to the mental and physical health, and may also increase chances of maternal mortality.

World Health Organization has defined unsafe abortion as an abortion not provided through approved facilities and/or persons.[16] These abortions, mainly in rural area, but also many times in urban area, are induced by patients themselves, or by nonmedical personnel or in unhygienic conditions. This is usually done by insertion of solid sticks/objects, or by consumption of various chemical agents, or by curettage with the use of unautoclaved instruments, leading to various critical complications like, hemorrhage, genital lacerations, perforation of uterus, tetanus, secondary infertility, chronic pelvic pain/infection, increased risk of ectopic pregnancy, and depression. Such patients are managed accordingly in form of initial resuscitation, broad spectrum antibiotics, SOS laparotomy for drainage of collection, and thorough curettage of uterine contents and tender psychological support.

Teenagers were found to be more distressed after abortions, as compared to adults undergoing abortions.[17]

With changing times, lifestyle modifications and career-oriented approach of females have led to later age of marriage with reduction in fertility in middle and higher socioeconomic class, but there has been yet lower age at marriage and increased fertility in lower socioeconomic class. From a larger global perspective, poorer countries have been facing issues in form of spread of human immunodeficiency virus (HIV) infection and lack of safe motherhood practices.

■ MAJOR HEALTH CONCERN

A teenage herself is at risk of having preexisting anemia and malnutrition, due to increasing demands and lack of adequate intake of nutrients. Growth of pelvic girdle succeeds long bone growth ending at around 18th year of age, thus making the former underdeveloped in teenage years.

Obstetric Complications

Pregnancy at the tender age of teenage has been associated with preterm delivery, perinatal morbidity and/or mortality, small for gestational age infants, maternal psychological disturbances, child's development, and growth along with life-long disability. The rate of low birth weight babies was double than that of adults. Neonatal mortality was almost three times than that delivered in adulthood. Maternal mortality was double than the rate during adult age group mothers.[18] Preterm delivery was found to be significantly higher in adolescent pregnancy as compared to adult mothers.[19] Birth defects were found to be higher in such pregnancies, than in age group of 20-30 years; neural tube defects were the most common.[20] These pregnancies have been found to be associated with increased chances of anemia, sexually transmitted infections (STIs), intrauterine growth restriction, preeclampsia, obstructed labor, postpartum hemorrhage, and puerperal sepsis. Birth injuries, vesicovaginal, and rectovaginal fistulae may be the outcome of avoiding institutional delivery due to social stigma. Non-to-so mature hormonal environment along with immaturity of gynecological organs and underdeveloped pelvis has contributed largely to these adverse outcomes.[21,22]

Mother and fetus both compete for nutrients, but preferred pathway of nutrients is always in favor of mother, who herself is in developing phase, depriving fetus of its essential requirements.[23] In a study conducted by Chaturvedi et al., diet of adolescent mothers were deficient in calories, proteins, iron and vitamin A, and 78% adolescent pregnant females were anemic.[24] In addition to improper nutrition, adolescent mothers are more likely to consume alcohol and smoking piling up the burden on mother as well as fetus. Smoking is also associated with additional risks of placental abruption, preterm birth, stillbirth, and sudden infant death.[25,26]

Lack of antenatal care was found to be one of the most important contributing factors toward adverse maternal and perinatal outcomes.[27]

Sexually Transmitted Infections

Mother to child transmission of HIV infection is of higher risk, as the infection would be recent one, with increased viral load. Coexisting STIs along with local infections and inflammation increases chances of baby getting infected during the process of labor. A study in USA concluded that 1 in 5 adolescent females had STI.[28]

Unsafe Abortions

Approximately 14% of unsafe abortions in low and middle-income countries occur in the age group of 15-19 years.[4]

Psychological, Social, and Academic Problems

Suicidal rates were also noted to be higher in teenagers who got married under 18 years of age, which in turn reflects hostile circumstances they had to live in.[29]

Adolescent pregnancy makes mothers leave their education, thus complicating the lives of family as a whole.[30] Such pregnancies would also impose as a burden on social and economic horizons of the society and country. Health indicators, i.e., maternal mortality rate, infant mortality rate, and abortion rates get worsen with teenage pregnancies.

Decision for termination of pregnancy is usually delayed due to late diagnosis of pregnancy, thus, more number of second trimester abortions, leading to more complications as compared to earlier abortions. Abortion, again, is a procedure "judged" by the society, making patient fail to report it as a part of past history.

Children Delivered from Adolescent Mothers

Nguyen concluded that first pregnancy in the age group of 10-19 years was associated with children with higher undernutrition risks, and significantly shorter in height than those born to adult mothers.[31] These mothers gradually face hardships in taking care of their children as well as themselves. First month of life for children delivered to adolescent mothers face almost 50-100% higher chances of deaths as compared to older mothers.

Children born of adolescent pregnancies struggle physically as well as psychologically. They face increased risk of academic underachievements, behavioral disturbances, substance abuse, and developmental delay.[32]

■ RESPONSIBLE FACTORS

Early marriage has been still a widespread practice in many developing countries. Expectation of the conception at the earliest after marriage has led to rise in adolescent mothers.

The age at menarche has fallen to an average of 12.8 years.[33] This has led to earlier sexual maturity and earlier child bearing in vulnerable scenario. Many a times, teenage mothers themselves were found to be result of teenage pregnancies.[34] In a study conducted in USA, approximately 56% of girls and 73% of boys had sexual intercourse before the age of 18 years.[35]

Physical/sexual abuse was again a major factor contributing to adolescent pregnancy. Approximately 50-60% of adolescent mothers reported to have had sexual abuse.[36] WHO data suggests around 20% of girls suffer from sexual abuse/violence in their childhood and adolescent phase.[37] Peer pressure in addition to other factors does play a major role in contributing to getting indulged in sexual practices.[38]

A study by Spitz et al. concluded that more than 90% of adolescent pregnancies were unintended.[39] Majorly, those teenagers who are homeless, who are forcefully thrown into roles of community sex workers, orphans, mentally/physically challenged, are the ones who are at risk of getting pregnant.

Girls belonging to families where fathers left in their early childhood, showed earlier sexual exposure, as compared to the ones where fathers stayed with family.

Media and exposure of children to explicit sexual content have also contributed significantly toward teenage pregnancy.[40] With advancing times, the age at first intercourse is on decline, and number of sexual partners before marriage is on rise!

Many barriers like lack of confidentiality, judgmental and untrained health providers, and cultural stigma prevent teenagers from approaching correct health advices.[41] As the girls below 18 years are minor, their parents need to be informed and consent needs to be taken from them, which again restricts the utilization of official services by teenagers on their own. Legally, parents are involved as minors are considered as incapable of making decisions, and parents on the other hand, are experienced, mature, and reasonable enough to make decisions, as well as to pay for the healthcare services. Parents also consider discussion about sexual relations as a taboo, which again closes the doors for teenagers.

Developing countries face a challenge of providing easy and free access to education, which in turn, encourage early and frequent childbearing with mentality of more income from more number of children.

MANAGEMENT OF TEENAGE PREGNANCY

Measures to abolish social exclusion, along with early access to the obstetric care, along with counseling, and various available options are essential for making a right choice followed by necessary medical and social measures. In developed countries, programs to educate such parents along with their societal rehabilitation have been implemented with huge success. Health clinics can serve youth with regards to contraceptive choices in a confident and nonjudgmental manner.

Prevention

England implemented "Teenage Pregnancy Strategy" in 1999 with the aims of reducing under 18 conception rate and reducing social exclusion by increasing education, training, and employment of these mothers.[42] The actions implemented were sex education and relationship counseling to positive and safe relationships, contraceptive practices, education about (STIs, and establishing communication with their parents.

Schools can help develop students physically, emotionally, and morally, along with sex education so as to make them responsible for their actions, along with making right choices based on knowledge rather than under peer pressure. Media can also play a major role in motivating teenage population.

A study conducted in UK concluded that teacher delivered program had great impact on students in form of reduced guilt and improvement in sexual health. Peer-delivered programs motivated youth to delay first intercourse.[42]

Values, responsibilities, and making right choices with confidence need to be taught, as a part of primary prevention. Such steps of primary prevention are found to be effective while maintaining confidence of youth, and preventing them to succumb to peer pressure. Nutritional status of teenagers needs to be focused on for overall health of future society.

Secondary prevention can be done by establishing clinics for teenagers for family planning. One idea is to notify parents of their teenagers so as to make them open up about sexual orientation and contraception, but it may back fire if the family follows strict no premarital sex.

Tertiary prevention is focused on managing teenage pregnant females, wherein prenatal counseling with various available options for termination of pregnancy, if that is possible, or measures for continuation of pregnancy with proper prenatal counseling can be explained. Healthcare services need to offer routine ultrasonography for estimation of gestational age and evaluation of growth of fetus. Early counseling helps in identification of risk factors. Information regarding pregnancy, modes of delivery, and counseling for child's care needs to be provided.

Delivery and Postpartum

Emotional support during labor process is preferred. Postpartum care is of importance, to make sure of full physical, psychological, and societal rehabilitation of the adolescent mother, along with proper care and upbringing of the child. Both parents need to be offered educational parenting classes and motivation and guidance for the care of family as a whole. Social and economic conditions of family, safety of newborn needs to be taken into account.

Adolescent mothers are shown to have breastfeeding difficulties, with approximately 37–54% reduction in milk production within first 6 months of childbirth, as compared to adult counterparts.[43]

Teenage parents usually lack self-esteem, self-efficiency, and they fail to empathize with others. Teenage parents need to be given support; so as to make them capable of personal and family's growth in right direction. They face social stigma and distressful reactions from family and friends leading to social isolation and depression.

Contraception

An adolescent, on an average takes approximately 12 months to seek contraceptive advice after becoming sexually active.[36] Oral and injectable contraceptives, barrier contraceptives are the ones which can be used by teenagers easily. Barrier contraceptives will additionally prevent STIs. They need to be given proper counseling and proper education about emergency contraceptive methods.

Community education in a multidisciplinary manner is recommended, including pediatricians, psychiatrists, gynecologists, and counselors, to encourage teenagers to use contraceptives, defer intercourse as late as possible, abstinence till the right time, and opening up about any fear/untoward incidents.

Those teenagers, who want to refrain from peer pressure of sex, need to be supported.

Netherlands showed a huge success by implementing curriculum focused on values, communication, attitude, along with support from media, and confidential healthcare system.[44]

World Health Assembly in May 2011 concluded specific measures including, protection of young people from early childbearing, access to contraception and healthcare facilities, access to accurate information of reproductive health, WHO published guidelines for middle and low-income countries, and implementation of guidelines prepared in association with United Nations Fund for Population Activities (UNFPA). Improved female literacy, opening opportunities for academics and vocational chances, and confidential and nonjudgmental counseling are the need on this hour to prevent and manage teenage pregnancies.

Adolescent health programs in India have been successfully implemented and have significantly contributed to improved health status of adolescents. Strict implementation of law for age at marriage is must to stop so called religious/cultural practices.

REFERENCES

1. UNFPA. Girlhood, not motherhood: preventing adolescent pregnancy. New York: UNFPA; 2015.
2. UNDESA. Population Division. World Population Prospects: The 2017 Revision. New York: UN DESA; 2017.
3. UNICEF. Ending child marriage: Progress and prospects. New York: UNICEF; 2013.
4. WHO. (2015). Maternal, newborn, child and adolescent health. [online] Available from: https://www.who.int/maternal_child_adolescent/en/ [Last accessed January, 2020].
5. WHO Maternal, newborn child and adolescent. Geneva: WHO Publication; 2012.
6. Wadhera S, Miller EJ. Teenage pregnancies 1974–1994. Health reports (Statistics Canada, Catalogue 82-003-XPB). Winker. 1997;9(3):1-13.
7. National Center for Health Statistics (2000). Technical appendix. Vital statistics of United States: Mortality. [online] Available from: www.cdc.gov/nchs/data/nvsr/nvsr48/nvs48_11:2000;48(3):100 [Last accessed January, 2020].
8. Hamilton BE, Ventura SJ, National center for health statistics (2012). Birth rates for US teenagers reach historic lows for all age and ethnic groups. [online] Available from: https://www.cdc.gov/nchs/products/databriefs/db89.htm [Last accessed January, 2020].
9. Guttmacher A. Eleven million teenagers-what can be done about the epidemic of adolescent pregnancies in the United States? New York: Alan Guttmacher Institute; 1976.
10. Sheel CN, Chhabra R. Introduction. In: Chhabra R, Nuna S (Eds). Abortion in India: an overview. New Delhi: Veerendra Printers; 1995. p. 4.
11. Chhabra R, Nuna SC. Abortion in India an overview. New Delhi: Veerendra Printers; 1995.
12. Greydanus DE, Senanayake P, Gains MJ. Reproductive health: an international perspective. Indian J Pediatr. 1999;66:415-24.
13. World Health Organization. Adolescent pregnancy: issues in adolescent health and development. Geneva: World Health Organization; 2004. p. 86.
14. International Institute for Population Sciences (2015–16). ICF National Family Health Survey (NFHS-4). [online] Available from: http://rchiips.org/nfhs/NFHS-4Reports/India.pdf [Last accessed January, 2020].
15. Darroch JE, Woog V, Bankole A, Ashford LS. Adding it up: Costs and benefits of meeting the contraceptive needs of adolescents. New York: Guttmacher Institute; 2016.
16. WHO/FHE/MSM/93-13. Abortion Frequency and mortality of unsafe abortions, 2nd edition. Geneva: WHO; 1993.
17. Franz W, Reardon D. Differential impact of abortion on adolescents and adults. Adolescence. 1992;27(105):161-72.
18. Davidson NW, Felice ME. Adolescent pregnancy. In: Friedman SB, Fisher M, Schonberg SK (Eds). Comprehensive Adolescent Health Care. St Louis, MO: Quality Medical Publishing Inc;1992. pp. 1026-40.
19. Centre for Disease Control and Prevention. Pregnancy, sexually transmitted disease and related risk behaviour among US adolescents. Atlanta GA: Centres for Disease Control and Prevention; 1994.
20. Russel JK. Early teenage pregnancy. Am J Obstet and Gynecol. 1982;3:1.
21. Lao TT, Ho LF. Relationship between preterm delivery and maternal height in teenage pregnancies. Hum Reprod. 2000;15:463-8.
22. Olausson PO, Cnattingius S, Haglund B. Does the increased risk of preterm delivery in teenagers persist in pregnancies after the teenage period? BJOG. 2001;108:721-5.
23. Scholl TO, Hediger ML, Scholl JI, Khoo CS, Fischer RL. Maternal growth during pregnancy and the competition for nutrients. Am J Clin Nutr. 1994;60:183-8.
24. Chaturvedi A, Kapil U, Barithi T, Gnanasekaran N, Pandey RM. Nutritional status of married adolescent girls in rural Rajasthan. Indian J Pediatr. 1994;61:695-701.
25. Scholl TO, Hediger ML. Weight gain, nutrition and pregnancy outcome findings from the Camden study of teenager and minority gravidas. Semin Perinatol. 1995;19:171-81.
26. Miller PM, Plant M. Drinking, smoking, and illicit drug use among 15 and 16 years old in United Kingdom. BMJ. 1996;313:394-7.
27. Bukulmez O, Deren O. Perinatal outcome in adolescent pregnancies: a case control study from a Turkish University Hospital. Eur J Obstet Gynecol Reprod Biol. 2000;88:207-12.
28. Weisenfeld HC, Lowry DL, Heine RP, Krohn MA, Bittner H, Kellinger K, et al. Self-collection of vaginal swabs for the

28. detection of *Chlamydia*, *Gonorrhoea*, and trichomoniasis: opportunity to encourage sexually transmitted disease testing among adolescents. Sex Transm Dis. 2001;28:321-5.
29. India State-Level Disease Burden Initiative Suicide Collaborators. Gender differentials and state variations in suicide deaths in India: the Global Burden of Disease Study 1990-2016. Lancet Public Health. 2018;3:E478-89.
30. World Bank. Economic impacts of child marriage: Global synthesis report. Washington, DC: World Bank; 2017.
31. Nguyen PH, Scott S, Neupane S, Tran LM, Menon P. Social, biological and programmatic factors link adolescent pregnancy to early childhood undernutrition: a path analysis of India's 2016 National Family and Health Survey. Lancet Child Adolesc Health. 2019;3(7):463-73.
32. Raunch-Elnekanco H. Teenage motherhood: its relationship to undetected learning problems. Adolescence. 1994;29(113):91-103.
33. Cabrera SM, Bright GM, Frane JW, Blethen SL, Lee PA. Age of thelarche and menarche in contemporary US females: a cross-sectional analysis. J Pediatr Endocrinol Metab. 2014;27(1-2):47-51.
34. Elfebein DS, Felice ME. Adolescent pregnancy. Pediatr Clin North Am. 2003;50:781-800.
35. Forrest JD. Timing of reproductive life stages. Obstet Gynecol. 1993;82:105-11.
36. Alan Guttmacher Institute. Sex and America's Teenagers. New York: NY Alan Guttmacher Institute; 1994.
37. WHO. Global and regional estimates on violence against women: Prevalence and health effects of intimate partner violence and non-partner sexual violence. Geneva: WHO; 2013.
38. The National campaign to prevent teen pregnancy (1997). What the polling data tell us: A summary of past surveys on teen pregnancy. [online] Available from: https://web.archive.org/web/20070223214706/http://www.teenpregnancy.org/resources/data/polling97.asp [Last accessed January, 2020].
39. Spitz AM, Velebil P, Koonin LM, Strauss LT, Goodman KA, Wingo P, et al. Pregnancy, abortion, and birth rates among US adolescents—1980, 1985, and 1990. JAMA. 1996;275:989-94.
40. L' Engle KL, Brown JD, Kenneavy K. The mass media are an important context for adolescents' sexual behaviour. J Adolesc Health. 2006;38(3):186-92.
41. Graham A. Contraceptive clinics for adolescents. IPPF Med Bull. 1998;32(3):4.
42. Baker P, Guthrie K, Hutchinson C, Kane R, Wellings K. Teenage pregnancy and reproductive health. Summary Review. London: RCOG; 2007.
43. Motil KJ, Kertz B, Thotathuchery M. Lactational performance of adolescent mothers shows preliminary differences from that of adult women. J Adolesc Health. 1997;20:442-9.
44. Guus V. "The Dutch Model". Paris: The UNESCO Courier; 2000.

CHAPTER 10

Anemia in Adolescents

Shilpa Singh, Bindiya Gupta

INTRODUCTION

Anemia refers to decrease in oxygen carrying capacity of blood due to reduced level of hemoglobin and red cell mass.[1] This leads to inability of body to meet its physiological needs. Anemia is defined as red blood cell mass or hemoglobin measurement less than two standard deviations below the mean for normal population.[2] It is a condition when the number of RBCs are below normal (<4.2 million/μL) or hemoglobin (Hb) level is <12 g/dL in women and <13 g/dL in men.[3] In children aged 6-14 years and adolescents 15-19 years cut off of Hb is <12 g/dL.

Anemia in adolescents limits learning ability, physical development, increases their vulnerability to infection, increases school dropout rates, and reduces physical fitness for various extracurricular activities. Apart from physical harm of anemia, deleterious socioeconomic effects have also been observed:
- Cost incurred by public and private sectors of therapeutic measures for anemia are huge
- Socially, burden of maternal morbidity and mortality are high
- Long-term harmful effect of impaired mental development.

ANEMIA THE GLOBAL BURDEN

Anemia is currently most common intractable nutritional problem in world that affects both developing and developed countries. According to WHO report adolescents, especially girls, have the highest prevalence of anemia between 12 and 15 years as they are vulnerable to iron deficiency due to increase in nutritional requirements. The overall prevalence of anemia in South-East Asia region, except Thailand, is more than 25% in adolescent girls while in some countries the prevalence is as high as 50%.[4]

As per WHO, around 2 billion people are anemic with 50% of all anemia attributed to iron deficiency and more than 89% of this burden occurred in developing countries.[5] UNICEF report states that there are approximately 2.5 cases of iron deficiency for each case of anemia. Although, iron deficiency anemia (IDA) is prevalent in all stages of life but is more prevalent in pregnant women and young children. As per WHO, 2002 report measures to address iron deficiency anemia are among most cost effective public health interventions.[6]

CAUSES OF ANEMIA IN ADOLESCENCE

Adolescents face high risk for iron deficiency anemia due to increased iron requirement, poor diet, chronic parasitic infections, and social evils like early marriage and adolescent pregnancy.[4]

Increased Iron Requirement

Adolescents face increased iron demand due to growth spurt which causes sharp increase in lean body mass, blood volume which in-turn cause increase in iron need for myoglobin in muscles and hemoglobin in blood. Peak age of increased iron requirement in girls is 14-15 and 15-17 years in boys.

The iron demand in pre-adolescent is 0.7-0.9 mg iron per day which increases to 1.4-3.2 mg/day in girls and 1.37-1.8 mg/day in boys.[7] Risk of iron deficiency subsides in boys after growth spurt but for girls menstruation starts 1 year after peak growth and iron requirement remains high throughout reproductive life. Monthly loss of iron is 12.5-15 mg/month or 0.5-0.9 mg iron per day. This continuous demand of iron needs to be met through iron supplements, food fortification or diet diversification.

Poor Adolescent Diet and Poor Bioavailability of Iron

In India, diet of girls aged between 13 and 18 years provides much lower iron than boys of same age. The factors responsible for poor dietary intake by these girls are:

- Social discrimination towards boys providing them better nutrition.
- Adolescents frequently consume snacks prepared from refined cereals and carbonated drinks with a lower inclination to eat fruit, vegetables, meat or other iron-rich foods. Girls consuming a vegetarian diet (45.8%) have more anemia prevalence than adolescents who have a mixed diet (30%).
- Adolescents, particularly those belonging to poor socioeconomic status have habit of consuming tea or coffee immediately after meals. This causes high concentration of inhibitors and poor concentration of enhancers.[8]
- Adolescent girls due to their dieting habit have a lower total intake of food.

Frequent Infections in Adolescence

In India, infectious diseases have high prevalence which increases iron requirement and increased chance of negative iron balance. Anemia is more common in adolescents with history of parasitic infections like hookworm as these infections disturb body's metabolism of iron, vitamins, and protein intake contributing to anemia.

Adolescent Pregnancy

Early marriage and pregnancy is a great menace for health of these young adolescent girls. Post marriage, there is a huge social pressure which results in early pregnancy and then these girls never come out of the vicious inter-generational cycle of anemia. In India, as per 2005–2006 data, 18.2% of girls are married by age 15 and 47.4% of girls are married by age 18.[1]

PRESENTATION OF ANEMIA IN ADOLESCENTS

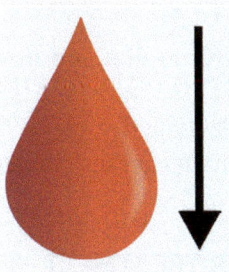

Pointers for anemia[2]
Anemia should be suspected in an adolescent, if there is:
- *Growth retardation:* Marked reduction in weight although height is unaffected. Onset of menses may also be delayed
- *Exercise intolerance:* Decrease in maximum work capacity and endurance
- *Behavioral changes:* Decreased attentiveness, poor memory, and school performance
- *Altered host response:* IDA affects both humoral as well as cell-mediated immunity

SIGNS AND SYMPTOMS OF ANEMIA

Anemia usually presents with nonspecific symptoms such as pallor, tiredness, lassitude, easy fatigability, weakness, and shortness of breath. It can be confused with respiratory illness, congestive cardiac failure (CCF), renal disease, and myxedema, so these conditions should be kept in mind when diagnosing anemia. Color of skin is not the best guide for severity of anemia as it depends on state of blood vessels in skin, amount of fluid in subcutaneous tissue, and on degree of skin pigmentation; hence, if pallor is out of proportion to actual anemia, nephrotic syndrome, hypoproteinemia, and CCF should be considered.[2]

PREVENTION OF ANEMIA IN ADOLESCENTS[1]

The strategies for prevention of anemia in adolescents are outlined in **Flowchart 1**.

Balanced Diet

Adolescence is very significant period for physical growth and sexual maturity. Eating a balanced diet, i.e., a diet that provides all nutrients (carbohydrate, protein, fat, vitamins and minerals) in required amounts and proportion is important for maintaining health and general well-being.

Foods which help in building up red cell mass are:
- Green vegetables and fruits
- Grains—wheat, jowar, bajra, sprouted pulse, groundnut, jaggery, and dry fruits
- Egg, fish, meat, milk products provide protein, i.e., body building food
- Vitamin C rich foods help in iron absorption—citrus fruit, amla, apple, pear

However, since it is not easy to change food habits or ensure access to iron rich foods, eating green vegetables appears to be only possible diet intervention even for low-income class. Green vegetables should be made essential part of mid-day meals and meals at *Anganwadi* centers.[9]

Iron Supplementation

As dietary interventions are not easy due to social factors and poverty, UNICEF and WHO proposed provision of universal iron supplements for adolescent girls[10,11] (especially those aged 12–16 years) and women of reproductive age group where anemia prevalence is greater than 20% in reproductive age group and greater than 40% among pregnant women. It is the optimum time to build

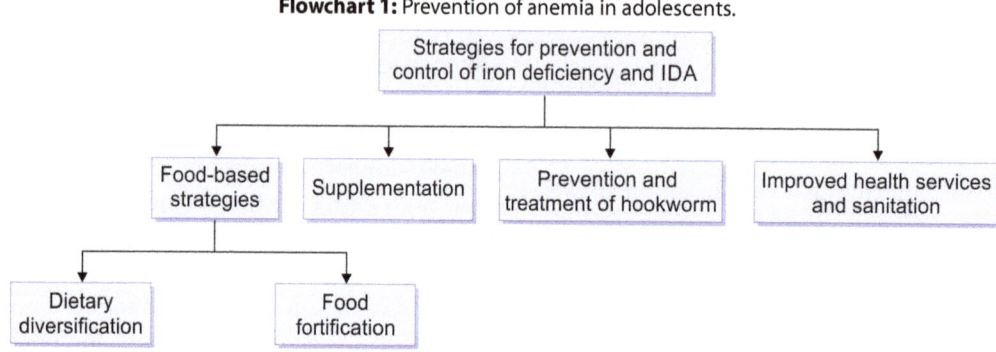

Flowchart 1: Prevention of anemia in adolescents.

(IDA: iron deficiency anemia)

iron stores before pregnancy. It has been found that iron supplementation at 10-14 years as compared to 15-18 years of age results in better weight gain[12] and menstrual cycle regulation.

Compliance to these daily iron supplementation programs is difficult due to nausea and medicinal iron after taste as well as poor health delivery systems. So, weekly consumption of one iron folic acid tablet (IFA) tablet containing 60 mg elemental iron and 2,800 μg folic acid[10,11] administered on a fixed day is proposed by Ministry of Health and Family Welfare–Govt. of India. It will be implemented in both rural and urban areas of India. Target population for weekly iron and folic acid supplementation (WIFS) program will be:

- *School based*: School-going adolescent girls and boys in government or government-aided schools from class VI to XII.
- *Community based*: Through *Anganwadi* centers aimed for out of school adolescent girls and adolescent pregnancy. Upon confirmation of pregnancy, WIFS should be replaced by daily 60 mg iron supplementation and 400 μg daily folic acid supplementation up till 3 months postpartum.

Advantages of weekly supplementation:
- It works as per mucosal block hypothesis according to which iron administration every 7 days allows time for shedding of iron loaded cells thereby increasing iron absorption.
- More efficacious approach in public health programs
- Cost effective
- Fewer side effects
- Ease of management at community level

For successful implementation of WIFS program, following issues should be addressed:
- Sustained political will
- Ensuring regular supply IFA tablets
- Using fixed weekly IFA day[13]
- Effective communication for generating willingness among participants to ingest them
- Innovative ways to ensure community participation including advertising in mass media
- Use of supplement record register and individual monitoring card to ensure compliance.

Prevention and Treatment of Hookworm

For prevention of hookworm infestation:
- Personal hygiene and sanitation should be maintained
- Clean water should be used for drinking and cooking food
- Avoidance of open air defecation, use of toilets, and washing hands properly after defecation as well as after discard fecal matter of child should be promoted
- Regular and proper hand washing practices before cooking or consuming foods should be practiced.

Soil transmitted helminths (STH) should be treated as per current WHO guidelines, i.e., if prevalence of STH in school-age children is >20% but <50%—tablet albendazole 400 mg once a year and if prevalence is >50% tablet albendazole 400 mg 6 monthly.[14]

Additional Interventions

Measures to combat anemia apart from diet and iron supplementation are:
- Use of iron fortified foods, e.g., salt, flour, rice, etc.
- Malaria prevention by use of mosquito's net and regular supply of insecticides.

■ THERAPEUTIC APPROACH FOR TREATMENT OF ANEMIA IN ADOLESCENTS

Screening

All in-school adolescents should be screened by teachers and out of school adolescents by anganwadi workers by

Table 1: Treatment and follow-up for management of anemia as per hemoglobin levels.

Level of Hb	Treatment	Follow-up
Mild anemia (11–11.9 g/dL)	60 mg of elemental iron daily for 3 months	Follow-up every month Hb estimation after completing 3 months of treatment to assess if Hb estimation are >12 g/dL
Moderate anemia (8–10.9 g/dL)	60 mg of elemental iron daily for 3 months	Investigate Follow-up every 14 days Hb estimation after completing 3 months of treatment to assess if Hb estimates are >12 g/dL
Severe anemia (<8 g/dL)	Refer urgently to first referral unit for further management and blood transfusion, if required	Severely anemic adolescents would be line listed by ANM

assessment of palms, nail bed, and tongue. Adolescents with clinical pallor should be referred to peripheral health centers (PHCs) for hemoglobin testing.[1]

After Hb testing at PHC, they will be categorized as having mild, moderate, and severe anemia on basis of hemoglobin levels and further management will be as described.

Management of Anemia as Per Hemoglobin Levels

The management of anemia as per hemoglobin levels is outline in **Table 1**.

Indications for blood transfusion in severe anemia:
- With Hb ≤4 g/dL
- With Hb 4–6 g/dL and presence of any one of following: dehydration, shock, impaired consciousness, heart failure, and labored breathing.

Injectable iron should be considered in cases if contraindication to oral therapy and patient is not compliant to take oral iron. The main advantage of parenteral therapy is certainty of its administration to correct Hb and fix-up iron stores.[15]

The non-responders of 3 month iron treatment should be investigated to determine cause of anemia that includes:
- Complete blood count
- Examination of peripheral blood smear
- Malaria parasite testing
- Stool examination for ova, cyst, and occult blood

CONCLUSION

Adolescence is the right time for interventions to address anemia. Iron is an essential nutrient required by body as it cannot be synthesized by body on its own. It has been rightly referred as body's gold which has to be built up to make a strong foundation for future.

REFERENCES

1. Adolescent Division, Ministry of Health and Family Welfare, Government of India. Guidelines for Control of Iron Deficiency Anaemia: National Iron+ Initiative. [online] Available from: https://nhm.gov.in/images/pdf/programmes/wifs/guidelines/Guidelines_for_Control_of_Iron_Deficiency_Anaemia.pdf. [Last accessed November, 2019.
2. Gupta P, Menon PSN, Ramji S, Lodha R. Approach to diagnosis of anemia. In: Gupta P (Ed). PG Textbook of Pediatrics, 2nd edition. New Delhi: Jaypee Brothers Medical Publishers (P) Ltd; 2018. p. 1515.
3. World Health Organization (2014). Global Nutrition Targets 2025: Anemia Policy Brief. [online] Available from: https://apps.who.int/iris/bitstream/handle/10665/148556/WHO_NMH_NHD_14.4_eng.pdf?ua=1. [Last accessed November, 2019].
4. World Health Organization. Prevention of Iron Deficiency Anemia in Adolescents. Role of Weekly Iron and Folic Acid Supplementation, 2011. [online] Available from: https://apps.who.int/iris/bitstream/handle/10665/205656/B4770.pdf?sequence=1&isAllowed=y. [Last accessed November, 2019].
5. Kassebaum NJ; GBD 2013 Anemia Collaborators. The global burden of anemia. Hematol Oncol Clin North Am. 2016;30:247-308.
6. World Health Organization (2002). The World Health Report 2002: Reducing risks, promoting healthy life. [online] Available from: https://www.who.int/whr/2002/en/whr02_en.pdf?ua=1. [Last accessed November, 2019].
7. Beard JL. Iron requirements in adolescent females. J Nutr. 2000;130(2S):440S.
8. International Institute for Population Sciences (IIPS) and ORC Macro. National family health survey (NFHS) III, 2005-06, India. Mumbai: IIPS, 2007. [online] Available from: https://dhsprogram.com/pubs/pdf/frind3/frind3-vol1andvol2.pdf. [Last accessed November, 2019].
9. Technical Handbook on Anaemia in Adolescents. Weekly iron and folic acid supplementation programme. [online] Available from: https://www.nhm.gov.in/images/pdf/programmes/wifs/guidelines/technical_handbook_on_anaemia.pdf. [Last accessed November, 2019].
10. World Health Organization, Regional Office for Western Pacific. Global consultation on weekly iron and folic acid supplementation (WIFS) for preventing anaemia in women of reproductive age, 25-27th April 2007. Manila: WHO-WPRO, 2007.

11. World Health Organization. Weekly iron and folic acid supplementation (WIFS) in women of reproductive age: its role in promoting optimal maternal and child health. Geneva: WHO, 2009.
12. Kanani S, Poojara RH. Supplementation with iron and folic acid enhances growth in adolescent Indian girls. J Nutr. 2000;130(2S):452S.
13. Khan NC, Thanh HT, Berger J, Hoa PT, Quang ND, Smitasiri S, et al. Community mobilization and social marketing to promote weekly iron-folic acid supplementation: a new approach toward controlling anaemia among women of reproductive age in Vietnam. Nutr Rev. 2005; 63(12 Pt 2):S87-94.
14. Action against worms. [online] Available from: https://mjmp.org/wp-content/uploads/2014/12/Action-Against-Worms-Newsletter-Aug-2007-WHO1.pdf. [Last accessed November, 2019].
15. Konar H. Medical and surgical illness complicating pregnancy. In: Konar H (Ed). DC Dutta's Textbook of Obstetrics, 7th edition. New Delhi: New Central Book Agency (P) Ltd.; 2011. pp. 260-305.

CHAPTER 11

Sexually Transmitted Infection in Adolescents

Suchitra N Pandit, Swati Bhargava

INTRODUCTION

Adolescents, defined by the World Health Organization (WHO) as persons between 10 years and 19 years of age (WHO), make up about 20% of the world's population, of whom 85% live in developing countries. Adolescence is a rather new concept historically, comprising a lengthy period of transition from childhood to adulthood, associated with an emerging awareness of sexuality and an age-specific drive to experiment with sex.

In many societies, the gap between the age of sexual maturity and that at which sexual relations become legitimate has widened.

Adolescence is commonly associated with physiological changes occurring with the progression from appearance of secondary sexual characteristics (puberty) to sexual and reproductive maturity (WHO).

Sexually transmitted infections (STIs) are infectious diseases spread through sexual contact. About 50 out of 100 new STIs happen in people ages 15–24 years.

Sexually transmitted diseases (STDs) are a serious health problem for adolescents, occurring in an estimated one-quarter of sexually active teenagers. Many of the health problems including STDs result from specific risk-taking behaviors. Determinants of STD risks among adolescents include behavioral, psychological, social, biological, and institutional factors. Education is an important component in STD control in adolescents. The goal of education is to increase adolescent self-efficiency in practicing STD prevention and risk reduction. A comprehensive approach including quality, theory-based education, accessible and effective health clinics, and improved social and economic conditions has the most promise of controlling STDs in adolescents.

Incidence and prevalence estimates suggest that young people aged 15–24 years acquire half of all new STDs[1] and that one in four sexually active adolescent females has an STD such as chlamydia or human papillomavirus (HPV).[2]

This age group (15–24 years) has increased susceptibility to infection because of increased cervical ectopy. Cervical ectopy refers to columnar cells, which are typically found within the cervical canal, located on the outer surface of the cervix. Although this is a normal finding in adolescent and young women, these cells are more susceptible to infection.

It may also reflect multiple barriers to accessing quality STD prevention and management services including inability to pay, lack of transportation, long waiting times, conflict between clinic hours and work and school schedules, embarrassment attached to seeking STD services, method of specimen collection, and concerns about confidentiality.

Sexually transmitted infections are on the rise possibly due to more sexually active people who have multiple sex partners during their lives.

Many STIs cause no symptoms at first and many STI symptoms may be confused with those of other diseases not spread by sex, especially in women. Even symptomless STIs can be contagious and can later cause long-term (chronic) or serious health problems.

The STIs may be the consequence of unprotected sex with a number of short-term partners, but may also occur among those who have a long-term unfaithful, perhaps older, partner or husband. Furthermore, for biological reasons, sexually active girls may be at greater risk of contracting STIs than boys. One of the reasons why young people are particularly vulnerable to STIs is the lack of sex education, including on STI prevention.

According to the WHO, 333 million new cases of curable STIs occur worldwide each year, with the highest rates among 20–24-year-old followed by 15–19-year-old (WHO).[3]

TYPES OF SEXUALLY TRANSMITTED INFECTIONS

- Chlamydia
- Gonorrhea
- Syphilis
- Hepatitis
- Herpes simplex
- Human immunodeficiency virus/acquired immunodeficiency syndrome (HIV/AIDS) and STDs
- Human papillomavirus (HPV) infection
- Pelvic inflammatory disease (PID)
- Bacterial vaginosis
- Trichomoniasis
- Other STDs—chancroid, scabies, cytomegalovirus, lymphogranuloma venereum, trichomoniasis, granuloma inguinale, etc.

Chlamydia

Infection with *Chlamydia trachomatis* (*C. trachomatis*) may result in urethritis, epididymitis, cervicitis, acute salpingitis, or other syndromes when sexually transmitted; however, the infection is often asymptomatic in women.

In 2017, a total of 1,708,569 cases of *C. trachomatis* infection were reported to the Centers for Disease Control and Prevention (CDC), making it the most common notifiable condition in the United States. This case count corresponds to a rate of 528.8 cases per 100,000 population, an increase of 6.9% compared with the rate in 2016. During 2016-2017, rates of reported chlamydia increased among both males and females in all regions of the United States and among all racial and Hispanic ethnicity groups.

Rates of reported chlamydia are highest among adolescent and young adults and have increased in recent years. In 2017, almost two-thirds of all reported chlamydia cases were among persons aged 15-24 years. Among women aged 15-24 years, the population targeted for chlamydia screening, the overall rate of reported cases of chlamydia, was 3,635.3 cases per 100,000 females, an increase of 4.9% from 2016 and of 8.8% from 2013.[4]

Although rates of reported cases among men are generally lower than rates among women, reflecting the larger number of women screened for this infection, rates among men increased almost 40% during 2013-2017. Increases in rates among men may reflect an increased number of men including gay, bisexual, and other men who have sex with men (collectively referred to as MSM) being tested and diagnosed with a chlamydial infection due to increased availability of urine testing and extragenital screening.[4]

Adolescents are believed to represent at least one-third of cases of *C. trachomatis* infection worldwide and perhaps an equal share of gonorrhea infection.[5,6]

In several studies, adolescent girls accounted for the highest level of chlamydial infection detected by culture among all age groups and among younger adolescents prevalence was higher than among older ones.[7]

Gonorrhea

The prevalence of gonorrhea among adolescent girls is usually lower than that of chlamydia.[8]

In 2017, a total of 555,608 cases of gonorrhea were reported to the CDC, making it the second most common notifiable condition in the United States. During 2016-2017, the rate of reported gonorrhea increased 19.3% among men and 17.8% among women. The magnitude of the increase among men suggests either increased transmission, increased case ascertainment (e.g., through increased extragenital screening among MSM), or both. The concurrent increase in cases reported among women suggests parallel increase in heterosexual transmission, increased screening among women, or both.

Coinfections and Sequelae

Chlamydia has been found to occur as a coinfection in patients treated for gonorrhea in up to 50% of cases, which has led the WHO to recommend that as a routine both infections should be treated simultaneously.

It leads to serious long-term sequelae including PID, ectopic pregnancy, and infertility.

Chlamydia infection may lead to "silent PID", i.e., when infertility occurs without any signs or symptoms. PID is most common in young women under 25 years of age and the risk of scarring of the fallopian tubes and infertility appears to increase with the number of episodes.[9]

Chlamydia and Gonorrhea among Adolescent Boys

Transmission rates between adolescent boys and girls were also found to be the same. Men get clinical symptoms that include purulent discharge and burning urination. Penile discharge, which is the main symptom of both chlamydia and gonorrhea, was the most frequent symptom mentioned.[10]

The acute and chronic consequences of chlamydia and gonorrhea in boys, including urethral stricture and prostatitis, are less severe than the sequelae in girls.

Chancroid

An STD characterized by painful genital ulceration and inflammatory inguinal adenopathy. The disease is caused by infection with *Haemophilus ducreyi*.

Syphilis

- Primary—a stage of infection with *Treponema pallidum* (*T. pallidum*) characterized by one or more ulcerative lesions (e.g., chancre), which might differ considerably in clinical appearance.
- Secondary—a stage of infection caused by *T. pallidum* characterized by localized or diffuse mucocutaneous lesions (e.g., rash—such as nonpruritic, macular, maculopapular, popular, or pustular lesions) often with generalized lymphadenopathy.

Syphilis seems to increase rather than to decrease with age and is therefore less a disease of adolescence than chlamydia and gonorrhea.[11]

Prevalence of syphilis of 5–8% has been found in several surveys among adolescents and young adults.[12,13]

Genital Herpes

A condition characterized by visible, painful genital or anal lesions. Herpes simplex virus-2 (HSV-2) is the most common cause of recurrent genital herpes among adolescents in developing countries.

Genital Warts

An infection characterized by the presence of visible, exophytic (raised) growths on the internal or external genitalia, perineum, or perianal region.

Granuloma Inguinale

A slowly progressive ulcerative disease of the skin and lymphatics of the genital and perianal area caused by infection with *Calymmatobacterium granulomatis*.

Lymphogranuloma Venereum

Infection with L1, L2, or, L3 serovars of *C. trachomatis* may result in a disease characterized by genital lesions, suppurative regional lymphadenopathy, or hemorrhagic proctitis. The infection is usually sexually transmitted.

Mucopurulent Cervicitis

Cervical inflammation that is not the result of infection with *Neisseria gonorrhoeae* (*N. gonorrhoeae*) or *Trichomonas vaginalis*. Cervical inflammation is defined by the presence of one of the following criteria:

- Mucopurulent secretion (from the endocervix) that is yellow or green when viewed on a white, cotton-tipped swab (positive swab test)
- Induced endocervical bleeding (bleeding when the first swab is placed in the endocervix).

Nongonococcal Urethritis

Urethral inflammation that is not the result of infection with *N. gonorrhoeae*. Urethral inflammation may be diagnosed by the presence of one of the following criteria:

- A visible abnormal urethral discharge
- A positive leukocyte esterase test from a male aged <60 years who does not have a history of kidney disease or bladder infection, prostate enlargement, urogenital anatomic anomaly, or recent urinary tract instrumentation
- Microscopic evidence of urethritis (≥ 5 white blood cells per high-power field) on a Gram stain of a urethral smear.

Pelvic Inflammatory Disease

A clinical syndrome resulting from the ascending spread of microorganisms from the vagina and endocervix to the endometrium, fallopian tubes, and/or contiguous structures.

Human Papillomavirus Infection

The prevalence of HPV, which initially manifests itself as genital warts, also seems to be higher among adolescents than adults, at least in developed countries.

■ BARRIERS TO EFFECTIVE SEXUALLY TRANSMITTED INFECTIONS CARE FOR ADOLESCENTS

- Barriers related to the asymptomatic nature of the most important infections and the lack of suitable methods to detect them
- Barriers related to adolescents' lack of knowledge about and awareness of the seriousness of STIs
- Most importantly, barriers in access to STI services including lack of availability of services and their cost.

The WHO has recommended the use of the "syndromic approach", which aims to enable healthcare workers to identify syndromes caused by one or more STIs on the basis of patients' complaints of symptoms, clinical signs, and risk assessments.[14]

- Inadequate sources of information and knowledge
- Lack of knowledge of STIs
- Adolescents lack awareness of the seriousness of STIs
- Shame, embarrassment, and failure to communicate about sexual health matters.

FACTORS PREVENTING ADOLESCENTS WITH SEXUALLY TRANSMITTED INFECTIONS FROM GETTING EFFECTIVE TREATMENT

Nature of Sexually Transmitted Infections and of Diagnostic Methods

- Infection often asymptomatic
- Lack of affordable screening tests
- Inaccurate risk assessments

Adolescents' Knowledge, Attitudes, and Skills Related to Sexually Transmitted Infections and Care-seeking

- Lack of knowledge of symptoms
- Sexually transmitted infection treatment is a low priority
- Do not know where to go for treatment
- Do not have the skills needed to express a sexual health problem
- Fear of examinations
- Fear of parents and other adults finding out.

Access to Services

- Long distances to clinics or lack of (money for) transport
- Inconvenient opening times for adolescents (e.g., clinic closed after school)
- Legal/policy restrictions (e.g., parental consent, need to bring partner)
- Unfriendly/judgmental providers
- High cost of treatment.

Poor Case Management

- Drug shortages
- Ineffective drugs or suboptimal doses used
- Failure of informal providers to educate, promote and offer condoms, and to notify partners.

CONSEQUENCES OF SEXUALLY TRANSMITTED INFECTIONS

- Some STIs can spread into the uterus and fallopian tubes and cause PID.
- It can lead to both infertility and ectopic (tubal) pregnancy.
- Some strains of HPV infection in women may also be linked to cervical cancer. In both women and men, these strains may cause anal, head, and neck cancer.
- Sexually transmitted infections can be passed from a mother to her baby before or during birth. It may cause congenital infections and later congenital malformations.

TREATMENT GUIDELINES (CENTERS FOR DISEASE CONTROL AND PREVENTION TREATMENT GUDELINES 2015)[15]

The recommended treatment guidelines according to the CDC are described in **Table 1**.

PREVENTIVE MEASURES

- Genital hygiene is essential.
- Avoiding intercourse prior to 18 years of age as it is restricted by law.
- Counseling for having safe sex practices at all ages.
- Have a mutually monogamous sexual relationship with an uninfected partner.
- Use (consistently and correctly) a male latex or female polyurethane condom, even for oral sex.
- Reduce chance of HIV infections by preventing and controlling other STIs. Having another STI makes it easier to get infected with HIV.
- Strongly think about HIV prevention treatments including:
  - Postexposure prophylaxis (PEP). Taking medicines to prevent HIV within 72 hours after a risky exposure
  - Preexposure prophylaxis (PrEP). Taking medicine regularly to prevent HIV infection if exposed at a future risky sexual contact.
- If you are going to have sex with someone who is HIV positive, be very sure the other person is taking their HIV medicines and that their viral load is completely under control (undetectable).
- Delay having sexual relationships as long as possible. The younger a person is when they start to have sex for the first time, the more susceptible they are to getting an STI.
- Have regular checkups for HIV and STIs.
- Learn the symptoms of STIs. Get medical help as soon as possible if you have any symptom.
- Do not have sex during menstruation.
- Do not have anal intercourse. Do not use a male latex condom and topical microbicides.
- Do not douche.

Table 1: Recommended treatment guidelines according to the CDC.

	Recommended treatment	Dose/route	Alternative
Bacterial vaginosis	Metronidazole oral[1] OR	500 mg orally 2×/day for 7 days	Tinidazole 2 g orally 1×/day for 2 days Or
	Metronidazole gel 0.75%[1] OR	One 5 g applicator intravaginally 1×/day for 5 days	Tinidazole 1 g orally 1×/day for 5 days Or Clindamycin 300 mg orally 2×/day for 7 days
	Clindamycin cream 2%[1,2]	One 5 g applicator intravaginally at bedtime for 7 days	Or Clindamycin ovules 100 mg intravaginally at bedtime for 3 days
Cervicitis	Azithromycin OR	1 g orally in a single dose	
	Doxycycline	100 mg orally 2×/day for 7 days	
Chlamydial infection	Azithromycin OR Doxycycline[4]	1 g orally in a single dose 100 mg orally 2×/day for 7 days	Erythromycin base 500 mg orally 4×/day for 7 days Erythromycin ethylsuccinate 800 mg orally 4×/day for 7 days Levofloxacin 500 mg 1×/day orally for 7 days Ofloxacin 300 mg orally 2×/day for 7 days
Epididymitis	Ceftriaxone Plus Doxycycline	250 mg IM in a single dose 100 mg orally 2×/day for 10 days	
Genital herpes simplex	Acyclovir OR	400 mg orally 3×/day for 7–10 days	
	Acyclovir OR	200 mg orally 5×/day for 7–10 days	
	Valacyclovir OR	1 g orally 2×/day for 7–10 days	
	Famciclovir	250 mg orally 3×/day for 7–10 days	
Genital warts (HPV)	Patient application: • Imiquimod 3.75% or 5% cream • Podofilox 0.5% solution or gel sinecatechins 15% ointment. Provider administered: • Cryotherapy • Trichloroacetic acid or bichloroacetic acid 80–90% • Surgical removal.		
Gonococcal infections	Ceftriaxone Plus	250 mg IM in a single dose	
	Azithromycin	1 g orally in a single dose	
Lymphogranuloma venereum	Doxycycline	100 mg orally 2×/day for 21 days	Erythromycin base 500 mg orally 4×/day for 21 days
Nongonococcal urethritis (NGU)	Azithromycin OR Doxycycline	1 g orally in a single dose 100 mg orally 2×/day for 7 days	
Pediculosis pubis	Permethrin 1% cream rinse OR Pyrethrins with piperonyl butoxide	Apply to affected area, wash off after 10 minutes	Malathion 0.5% lotion, applied 8–12 hours then washed off Or Ivermectin 250 μg/kg orally, repeated in 2 weeks

Contd...

Contd...

	Recommended treatment	Dose/route	Alternative
PID	*Parenteral regimens:* Cefotetan Plus Doxycycline Cefoxitin Plus Doxycycline *Recommended intramuscular/ oral regimens:* Ceftriaxone Plus Doxycycline with or without metronidazole OR Cefoxitin Plus Probenecid Plus Doxycycline with or without metronidazole	2 g IV every 12 hours 100 mg oral or IV 12 hourly 2 g IV every 6 hours 100 mg oral or IV 12 hourly 250 mg IM in a single dose 100 mg oral BD for 14 days 500 mg oral BD for 14 days 2 g IM in single dose 1 g oral 100 mg oral BD × 14 days 500mg oral BD × 14 days	*Parenteral regimens:* Ampicillin/Sulbactam 3 g IV every 6 hours PLUS Doxycycline 100 mg orally or IV every 12 hours
Scabies	Permethrin 5% cream OR Ivermectin	Apply to all areas of body from neck down, wash off after 8–14 hours 200 μg/kg orally, repeated in 2 weeks	Lindane 1% 1 oz. of lotion or 30 g of cream, applied thinly to all areas of the body from the neck down, and wash off after 8 hours
Syphilis	Benzathine penicillin G	2.4 million units IM in single dose	Doxycycline 100 mg 2×/day for 14 days Tetracycline 500 mg orally 4×/day for 14 days
Trichomoniasis	Metronidazole OR Tinidazole Metronidazole If regimen fails: Metronidazonle OR Tinidazole	2 g oral in single dose 2 g oral in single dose 500 mg oral 2×/day for 7 days 2 g oral for 7 days 2 g oral for 7 days	Metronidazole 500 mg 2×/day for 7 days

(CDC: Centers for Disease Control and Prevention; HPV: human papillomavirus; IM: intramuscular; IV: intravenous; PID: pelvic inflammatory disease)

REFERENCES

1. Satterwhite CL, Torrone E, Meites E, Dunne EF. Sexually transmitted infections among US women and men: Prevalence and incidence estimates, 2008. Sex Trans Dis. 2013;40:187-93.
2. Forhan SE, Gottlieb SL, Sternberg MR, Xu F, Datta SD, McQuillan GM, et al. Prevalence of sexually transmitted infections among female adolescents aged 14 to 19 in the United States. Pediatrics. 2009;124:1505-12.
3. World Health Organization. Press release, WHO/64. Geneva: World Health Organization; 1995.
4. Workowski KA, Bolan GA, Centers for Disease Control and Prevention. Sexually transmitted diseases treatment guidelines, 2015. MMWR Recomm Rep. 2015;64:1-137.
5. Cates W, Mc Pheeters. Adolescents and Sexually Transmitted Diseases: Current Risks and Future Consequences. Paper Prepared for the Workshop on Adolescent Sexuality and Reproductive Health in Developing Countries: Trend and Interventions. Washington: National Research Council; 1997.
6. Senderowitz J. Health Facility Programs on Reproductive Health for Young Adults. Washington: Focus on Young Adults Research Series; 1997.

7. Brabin L, Kemp J, Obunge OK, Ikimalo J, Dollimore N, Odu NN, et al. Reproductive tract infections and abortion among adolescent girls in rural Nigeria. Lancet. 1995;345:300-4.
8. Blankhart D, Müller O, Gresenguet G, Weis P. Sexually transmitted infections in young pregnant women in Bangui, Central African Republic. Int J STD AIDS. 1999;10:609-14.
9. Martin DH. Chlamydial infections. Med Clin North Am. 1990;74:1367-87.
10. Zambia. (1996). Demographic and Health Survey. [online] Available from: https://www.dhsprogram.com/pubs/pdf/FR86/FR86.pdf. [Last accessed April, 2020].
11. Hughes J, Berkley S. Convergence in Contexts and Opportunities for Research: STDs among Adolescents in Developing and Developed Countries. New York: The Rockefeller Foundation and International AIDS Vaccine Initiative; 1999.
12. Harms G, Iyambo SN, Corea A, Radebe F, Fehler HG, Ballard RC. Perceptions and patterns of reproductive tract infections in a young rural population in North-West Namibia. Int J STD AIDS. 1998;9:744-50.
13. Blankhart DM. Evaluation du project jeunes pour jeunes de l´ABBEF Ouagadougou, Burkina Faso. Ouagadougou: ABBEF; 1997.
14. World Health Organization. Report of the WHO Commissioned Studies on the Provision of Reproductive Health Services to Adolescents in Indonesia, Nigeria, and the Philippines. Geneva: World Health Organization; 1995.
15. Centers for Disease Control and Prevention (CDC). (2015). 2015 Sexually Transmitted Diseases Treatment Guidelines. [online] Available from: https://www.cdc.gov/std/tg2015/default.htm. [Last accessed April, 2020].

CHAPTER 12

Contraception in Adolescents

Girish Mane, Santosh Maid

INTRODUCTION

As a gynecologist, shall we advice contraception to the adolescents is a big question. Ideally, abstinence is the best contraception for all adolescents. Adolescent age starts from 12 years up to 25 years. As we all know, Government of India has implemented a new act to handle the sexual abuse against any person below 18 years which is known as the Protection of Children from Sexual Offences (POCSO) Act, 2012, which says that every person who has knowledge or has apprehension about the sexual abuse or activity against anyone below 18 years shall inform the local police or Special Juvenile Police Unit (SJPU) immediately. If failed to inform, the person is punishable for imprisonment and obviously the person performing or attempting the abuse or activity is also punishable strictly.

It means that government is very keen to protect the adolescents below 18 years of age from sexual abuse and sexual activity, even if the sexual act is consented by the girl. So with this situation, it is a big controversy about advising as well as providing the contraception to the girls below age of 18 years. It is an encouragement for sexual activity that is a personal view for every clinician, but magnitude of the problems arising in the adolescent age group is rising day-by-day to very alarming situation because of the lack of knowledge and use of contraception. It is said that the least age of loss of virginity in metro cities is 14 years in India. The average premature and premarital sexual involvement of girls in India is around 60% presently. Along with the self-premature sexual involvement of adolescent girls, the sexual abuse in India is rising day-by-day to the dangerous levels.

There are many factors pushing the adolescents toward premature or premarital sexual involvement in the current era like:
- Social media with easy internet availability
- No control on the net usability
- Effect of changed films and television culture
- Peer pressure
- Increased substance abuse in youngsters
- Wrong idols in youngsters
- Effect of western culture
- Small family norms and nuclear family
- Miscellaneous reasons.

These are the complications or problems because of unprotected sexual activity which can put the adolescents in extreme danger.
- Sexually transmitted diseases (STDs)
- Human immunodeficiency virus (HIV)
- Pelvic inflammatory disease (PID)
- Teenage pregnancies with complications like hypertensive disorders of pregnancy (HDP), premature deliveries, and antepartum hemorrhage (APH)
- Teenage unsafe abortions
- Teenage deliveries with increased instrumental or surgical deliveries, postpartum hemorrhage (PPH)
- Future subfertility or infertility because of PID or complications of abortions
- Mortality because of teenage abortions, pregnancies, and deliveries.

To prescribe the contraceptives to the girls below 18 years may not be parallel to the law, but it is the need of time to educate as well as to provide the contraception to the girls above 18 years.

BEST PRACTICES IN PRESCRIBING CONTRACEPTION

More holistic approach is needed while prescribing the contraception to the adolescents. One should explore the personal factors, psychosocial circumstances, and thorough sexual health history of the adolescent. Along with it, screening for pregnancy and sexually transmitted infections (STIs) or other associated health issues should be looked for. Promote abstinence if possible or safer sex practices and explain suitable contraceptive option. In fact, we should provide them the details of each and every method of contraception with their details and ask them to choose according to their circumstances and no doubt as a healthcare provider our input is must. Along with this, they should be provided the knowledge about the POCSO Act, 2012.

In this task, as a healthcare provider, one may face the challenges like the attitude of adolescent to confidentiality, accessibility, and affordability of methods. There can be barriers in communication as well as geographical difficulties for those in rural and regional areas. The counseling should differ between early, middle, and late adolescent females according to their contraceptive needs. If needed, both partners should be counseled together rather it is always beneficial. The final goal of this task is to prevent the adolescent girl from STIs and unwanted pregnancy and its complications.

The options of contraception are:
- Abstinence
- Barrier contraception
- Combined oral contraceptive pill (COCP)
- Long-acting reversible contraceptives (LARCs)
- Emergency contraception
- Other methods.

Abstinence

Even though it is difficult and none of our business to explain, advice, and force the adolescents for abstinence, one should have holistic approach in this regard. The girl cannot talk in this aspect with parents or teachers, but she is comfortable as well as believe in her doctor. She may not be aware of all sides of this act, so proper counseling may divert her thoughts and she may adapt abstinence which is the best, cheapest, most protective, and use full contraception in many regard. Also, if the girl is below 18 years of age, both the partners should be made aware of the POCSO Act, 2012 in detail.

Barrier Contraception

If the couple is not ready for abstinence, then it is the duty of the healthcare provider to proceed with due respect to their choice. Male condom is the most common, well-accepted, and effective type of barrier contraception. There are other options like diaphragm, cervical cup, sponge, and female condom too, but it is always wise to advice the male type in this age group. It has many advantages like easy availability, easy to use, and affordability. Also, it is available in nonmedical shops and does not need prescription of doctor.

Also, it has a special advantage of protection against STIs and HIV which should be the target for adolescent age group. So, practically if any girl is using or preferring other contraception, additional use of barrier contraception is always wise, but if the couple is in loyal relationship, then should be treated as adult or married couple, provided they are above 18 years of age. The only big problem of the male condom is that the failure rates in adolescents are higher than adults. May be it is due to the difficulty in correct and timely use. This difference may be because of difference in experience as well as size of their bodies. Failure rates can range as high as 13 pregnancies per 100 users. Other disadvantages are complaints of decreased sexual pleasure, itching, irritation on genitalia or sometimes burning, and micturition. So, the advice for the use of emergency contraception should be pass on after the tear or slipped off condom by adolescent male.

Combined Oral Contraceptive Pill

For the couple in long-term loyal relation and the girl with the abnormal uterine bleeding (AUB) or polycystic ovary syndrome (PCOS), COCP is an effective method. It prevents pregnancy through inhibition of ovulation and thickening of cervical mucus. COCP also provides multiple gynecological benefits in the form of menstrual cycle regulation, reduction of dysmenorrhea and heavy menstrual bleeding, and improving acne and hirsutism. However, the failure rate is high in adolescent age group due to the compliance challenges associated with daily administration reporting six to eight pregnancies per 100 women in the first 12 months of use. There can be discontinuation of contraceptive pills commonly due to irregular bleeding in the first few months of use. Other common side effects are vomiting, headache, nausea, and breast tenderness. There are many combinations of the COCP available with target-specific goals such as weight, acne, and hirsutism which can be chosen according to the need. In the girls with PCOS, the COCP with antiandrogen progesterone like drospirenone, desogestrel should be preferred.

Long-acting Reversible Contraceptives

The examples of LARC are intrauterine devices (Copper T, Multiload, and levonorgestrel intrauterine system, e.g., Emily, Mirena), the Implanon implantable device, and the injectable contraception.

The facts about LARC are:
- >99% effective
- 100% reversible
- <5% adolescents on globe use it

- <1% risk of complication
- 10% is rate of discontinuation
- 1/1,000 rate of perforation by intrauterine contraceptive device (IUCD) or intrauterine system (IUS).

Intrauterine contraceptive device is safe, effective, convenient, reversible, long acting, cost-effective, and easy to use method for contraception in females. If adolescents are in active sexual practice with a single partner, then this can be a good option for her. It is available as Copper T 380, Copper T 220C, the Multiload Copper T 375, and Nova T. There are few contraindications, few side effects, and rare complications with IUCD. The major disadvantage is that it does not protect from STIs, but the list of advantages is longer than disadvantages. The failure rate is extremely less than barrier or COCP.

Levonorgestrel intrauterine system is a very effective form of contraception releasing levonorgestrel continuously over a period of 5 years. Contrary to perceptions regarding its use, the IUS is a safe method for adolescents and has a low failure rate of 0.8 pregnancies per 100 women in the first 12 months of use. The IUS can safely be inserted in the small setting and importantly, in adolescents, there is no increased risk of insertion complications such as uterine perforation. The risk of pelvic infection following insertion is minimal due to the protective effect of cervical mucus, but it does not prevent the STIs. Use of IUS is very less in India as compared to the western countries.

The Implanon implantable device is another type of LARC. It is a flexible plastic rod about the size of 4 cm, inserted in the inner upper arm, which releases progesterone continuously for 3 years. The failure rate is very low at 0.1 pregnancies per 100 women. Its high effectiveness, action for long duration, and easy compliance for the user are the major advantages. One of the major disadvantages, however, is irregular vaginal bleeding, usually within the first 3–6 months following insertion, which can disturb the adolescents from its use and no protection from STIs.

The injectable contraception (Depo-Provera) contains medroxyprogesterone acetate (MPA) and is given every 3 months. It is an effective form of contraception. Its failure rate varies between one and eight pregnancies per 100 women due to noncompliance with repeating the injection typically in adolescent age group. Irregular bleeding pattern is one of the major side effects, which have been reported to be as high as in 30% users. There can also be a delay in the return of fertility from the last injection and loss of bone mineral density with long-term use, which does resolve once discontinued and it does not provide protection from STIs.

Emergency Contraception

This should be the choice of contraception in the immediate time period following unprotected sexual intercourse to prevent pregnancy. There are various options available like selective progesterone receptor modulator (ulipristal acetate), levonorgestrel, and high-dose combined pill (Yuzpe) as well as the intrauterine copper device insertion. Ulipristal acetate has proven higher efficacy than the other methods, especially if taken within the first 24 hours of unprotected sexual intercourse and is effective for up to 5 days. On the other hand, levonorgestrel-only regimen will prevent 85% of pregnancies up to 3 days after unprotected sexual intercourse and Yuzpe will prevent up to 75%. There are few side effects of these methods due to the high dose of hormones in their composition, which can alter the bioavailability of the drug. These effects are only transitory. There is no issues of return of fertility rather the fertility return is immediate and therefore a long-term treatment plan with the adolescent must be initiated. Alternatively, the copper intrauterine device can be inserted up to 5 days following unprotected sexual intercourse and has the added advantage of long-term contraception. Access to emergency contraception is just as important as the efficacy of these methods, as the success will decrease with time elapsed from unprotected sexual intercourse. Healthcare provider should educate the adolescents about the different methods available and how to source them. Pregnancy status must also be checked 3–4 weeks after initiation to verify success of treatment.

Other Options

There are a variety of other contraceptive methods available like natural methods. It is classified as:
- Fertility awareness method
- Periodic abstinence method
- Withdrawal method or coitus interruptus.

Practically, these are less suitable to the adolescent group. The failure rate will be very higher in these techniques. Also, the protection against the STIs will be zero and as this age group is not aware of the menstrual physiology and is usually facing the menstrual abnormalities, it is difficult for them to follow the menstrual calendar. Periodic abstinence and withdrawal techniques are very difficult to be followed by adolescent age group.

■ CONCLUSION

Contraception in adolescents is an important and controversial topic practice upon. We as a clinician are aware of the fact that it is almost impossible to stop the premarital sexual involvement in adolescents. We should think of the disasters happening because of it. Probably, the answer for these disasters is the provision of proper contraceptive majors and as gynecologists, we must consider the entire clinical picture when approaching each individual to ensure the most suited method for contraception. Once the contraception plan has been established, a follow-up appointment should be made within 3 months as a responsible healthcare provider. This practice will help to monitor and ensure correct use of contraception as well as confirming that the adolescent is satisfied with every type of outcomes and while prescribing contraception to the girl below the age of 18 years, you should be well aware of the POCSO Act, 2012, which says that "any person who has knowledge or apprehension about the sexual act performed or likely to be performed with or without consent of a girl below 18 years, they should inform the SJPU or local police about it without any delay. If fails to do so, you are punishable for the imprisonment for 6 months".

CHAPTER 13

Sexual Reproductive and Health Rights in Adolescents

Rohan Palshetkar, Jiteeka Thakkar

INTRODUCTION

The onset of adolescence not only brings changes to the body of young adults but also new vulnerabilities to human right abuse especially in arenas of sexuality, marriage, and childbearing. Many adolescents are coerced into unwanted sex or marriage, putting them at risk of unwanted pregnancies, unsafe abortions, sexually transmitted infections (STIs), and dangerous childbirth. Yet there are too many adolescents that face barriers to reproductive health information and care. Even those able to find accurate information about their health and rights may be unable to access the services needed to protect their health.

Sexual and reproductive health (SRH) is an essential component of the universal right to the highest attainable standard of physical and mental health. This has been included in the Universal Declaration of Human Rights and in other international human rights conventions. SRH includes both men and women.

Sexual and reproductive health rights (SRHR) include access to basic sexual and reproductive healthcare and information as well as autonomy in sexual and reproductive decision making. It allows both men and women to have the right to a healthy, safe, consensual, and enjoyable sex life. It allows them to have information to make decisions and seek healthy behavior. It also gives them access to affordable and accessible services that not only keep them healthy during pregnancy but also before and after, and even if they choose not to get pregnant.

Sexual and reproductive health rights are most clearly defined in the 1994 International Conference on Population and Development (ICPD) Programme of Action, which took place in Cairo, Egypt. Among the elements of comprehensive SRHR outlined in the Programme of Action are:
- Voluntary, informed, and affordable family planning services
- Pre-natal care, safe motherhood services, assisted childbirth from a trained attendant (e.g., a physician or midwife), and comprehensive infant healthcare
- Prevention and treatment of STIs, including human immunodeficiency virus and acquired immunodeficiency syndrome and cervical cancer
- Prevention and treatment of violence against women and girls, including torture
- Safe and accessible post-abortion care and, where legal, access to safe abortion services
- Sexual health information, education, and counseling, to enhance personal relationships and quality of life.

What does it take to meet the right to SRH?
In addition to identifying critical components of SRH, the ICPD Programme of Action makes recommendations for ensuring these rights are met, including:
- Freedom from discrimination
- Universal access to education
- Control of one's fertility, including the choice of whether and when to marry or have children, and protection from forced sterilization
- Protection of the family structure, with the understanding that there is a great diversity of family structures that are equally deserving of respect and safeguarding
- Recognition in policy and practice of the links between SRH, development, and the environment
- Prevention of early or forced marriage and inclusion of adolescents in planning and implementation of services and programs
- Engagement of men and boys
- Respect of the sexual orientation and gender identity of all individuals; and
- Full funding at the national and global levels to ensure universal access to basic healthcare, including SRH.

GENDER EQUALITY AND SEXUAL AND REPRODUCTIVE HEALTH RIGHTS

Sexual and reproductive health rights cannot be achieved without gender equality and woman's rights. In India, where most of the families are patriarchal, women tend to be financially dependent on their spouse and this can cause discrepancy in SRHR. Women are disproportionately affected by poverty, violence, a lack of access to decision-making and political processes, and low social status, all of which arise from gender-based discrimination and lead to disproportionate human rights abuses, including of the right to health. Pregnancy seems to be the only thing linked to reproductive health and therefore, women face major hurdles in attaining high standards of health. Women are sometimes valued only as incubators, therefore making them more vulnerable to human right abuses as they are valued less than men. Moreover, reproductive capacity of women may be used as a tool for abuse ranging from domestic violence to genocide.

Menstrual Hygiene

Menstruation is a process which every adolescent woman goes through. Unfortunately, in India, it is considered a major taboo. Women are ostracized during their menstrual cycle. This backward tradition is still very prevalent in many parts of the country. A lot of women are still using cloth in place of a sanitary pad which leads to sepsis and sometimes may even lead to the death of the women. Due to this, even a movie (PADMAN) based on menstrual hygiene was released in order to bring about the awareness of availability of economical, indigenous, hygienic, and environmentally sustainable methods of managing menstruation and also to reduce the taboo surrounding it. It is encouraging to see Akshay Kumar, one of the stars of Indian Cinema, bringing this into fruition. FOGSI tied up with Niine Foundation to bring about awareness by having the Run4Niine program on 8th March (Women's Day).

Adolescent Health

The age of onset of sexual intercourse has drastically decreased in the past decade or so. The average age of onset of intercourse in India is 15–18 years of age. The availability of contraception is a must in this age group. Introduction of adolescent friendly health services and cafeteria approach is an excellent method to provide adolescents with various contraceptive choices. Due to a decreasing age of onset of sexual intercourse, risk of STIs is high and therefore, reduction in STIs is a must. Sex education is a vital component of SRH in bringing about awareness. Sex education needs to be introduced into the system in an age appropriate manner in order to give the right information to adolescents in order for them to make informed choices regarding their sexual behavior. Counseling regarding use of condoms and reducing the number of sexual partners is necessary especially in the adolescent age group. Interventions using mass media campaigns can bring about awareness. Besides preventing STIs and treating them, access to safe abortion is also a woman's SRHR. It is a woman's choice whether to get pregnant or not, irrespective of her marital status. In India, even now, intercourse prior to marriage is considered a taboo. Hence, parents of minors or women who are unmarried may carry out unsafe marriages to try and hide the pregnancy.

Even now, over 14% of women get married under the age of 18 in India. In 1994, India employed a program called Apni Beti, Apna Dhan to incentivize the prevention of child marriage. However, such interventions where financial incentives are involved were difficult to sustain. Educating the general public about the harm of early onset of sexual intercourse and adolescent pregnancy would help in reducing this problem.

Right to Choose a Partner

The right to choose a partner is fundamental aspect of reproductive health. It is up to oneself to choose a partner not only for sexual gratification but also for mental peace. Even if it is a partner of the same sex, it is the right of an individual to decide. Till 2018, due to IPC 377, homosexuality was criminalized in India. A Supreme Court decision on September 6, 2018 decriminalized Section 377 of IPC and allowed gay sex among consenting individuals. Since now it is legalized, same sex couples deserve the same SRHR as heterosexual couples. Besides this, healthcare providers need to be more sensitive regarding the special needs of same sex couple.

This article is to bring about the awareness of Sexual Reproductive Health Rights for adolescents. So how can we bring about changes? Who can we turn in order to protect these rights? If a man or woman approaches, figures of authority, they should be treated with great sensitivity. Figures, who are in authority, have a responsibility to fight for and protect these rights. As gynecologists, we should be more sensitive towards adolescents, and ensure we protect their sexual reproductive health rights. Besides this, we should involve adolescents themselves in sexual reproductive health right programs and policies. It is important that they are able to voice their needs, realities, and opinions. By involving them, they will gain knowledge regarding SRHR programs which enables them to make informed decisions regarding their sexual health and rights.

CHAPTER 14

The Protection of Children from Sexual Offences Act, 2012 (POCSO): What Every OB-GYN Specialist should Know?

MC Patel, Manish Machave

Ignorantia juris non excusat (Ignorance of Law is no Excuse)

INTRODUCTION

Violence against children in India is a growing concern with mind boggling statistics. One out of every ten women reported some kind of child sexual abuse during childhood, chiefly by known persons. 1 out of 4 girls is sexually abused before the age of 4, 19% are abused between the ages of 4 and 8, 28% are abused between the ages of 8 and 12 and 35% are abused between the ages of 12 and 16.

There are approximately 2 million children commercial sex workers between the age of 5 and 15 years and about 3.3 million between 15 and 18 years. The children form 40% of the total population of commercial sex workers in India of which 80% of these are found in the 5 metros, 71% of them are illiterate and around 500,000 children are forced into this trade every year.

Provisions existing under the Indian Penal code, 1860 are Rape-Sec. 375/376 IPC, Kidnapping-Sec. 363-373 IPC, Molestation-Sec. 354 IPC and Sexual Harassment-Sec. 509 IPC, but all fall short to counter this menace of child sexual abuse.

NEED AND PURPOSE OF THE POCSO ACT 2012

To deal with child sexual abuse cases, the Government has brought in a special law, namely, The Protection of Children from Sexual Offences (POCSO) Act, 2012. The Act has come into force with effect from 14th November, 2012 along with the rules framed thereunder. The POCSO Act, 2012 is a comprehensive law to provide for the protection of children from the offences of sexual assault, sexual harassment and pornography, while safeguarding the interests of the child at every stage of the judicial process by incorporating child-friendly mechanisms for reporting, recording of evidence, investigation and speedy trial of offences through designated special courts.

The existing laws (IPC, IT Act, 2000 and JJ Act, 2000) not enough to address sexual offences, and also, there exist no specific provisions or laws for dealing with sexual abuse of male children.

This act provides protection to all children from the offences of sexual assault, sexual harassment, and pornography wherein a child is defined as any person below the age of 18 years.

SALIENT FEATURES OF THE POCSO ACT 2012

The act provides provisions for new offences/special courts/special public prosecutor. It also entails mandatory reporting/punishment for false reporting, special procedures for recording of complaint, statements and evidence, creation and monitoring by National Commission for Protection of Children's Rights (NCPCR), State Commission for Protection of Children's Right (SCPCR), Convergence with The Juvenile Justice Act 2000, and provisions for monetary compensation of the victim.

APPLICABILITY OF THE POCSO ACT

The POCSO Act is gender neutral. Sexual offences in the IPC are gender specific. The provisions (with the exception of Section 377) only apply to women as victims, while the perpetrators are male. In contrast, the POCSO Act protects children of both sexes from sexual offences and is only applicable to child survivors and adult offenders.

In case two children have sexual relations with each other, or in case a child perpetrates a sexual offence on an adult, the Juvenile Justice (Care and Protection of Children) Act, 2000, shall apply.

OFFENCES AND PUNISHMENTS UNDER THE ACT

All offences under the act are cognizable (arrest without warrant) and nonbailable (No bail as a right).

There are various offences defined and punished under The POCSO Act 2012, Penetrative Sexual Assault (Sec. 3), Aggravated Penetrative Sexual Assault (Sec. 5), Sexual Assault (Sec. 7), Aggravated Sexual Assault (Sec. 9), and Sexual Harassment (Sec. 11).

Rigorous punishments for offenders are defined in the act. Section-4-Imprisonment up to 3 years and also liable to fine not less than 3 years but may extend to 5 years and also liable to fine, Section-6-Not less than 7 years, may extend to imprisonment for life and also liable to fine, Section-8 Not less than 5 years, may extend to 7 years and also liable to fine, Section-10-Rigorous Imprisonment for not less than 10 years, may extend to imprisonment for life, also liable to fine, using a child for pornographic purposes [Section 14 (1)]: Up to 5 years and fine.

Using a child for pornographic purposes, after having been convicted previously for same offence [Section 14 (1)]: Up to 7 years imprisonment and fine. Storing, for commercial purpose, any pornographic material in any form involving a child (Section 15): Up to 3 years or fine or both.

Attempting to commit any offence under this act (Section 18): One-half of the longest term of imprisonment provided for that offence with fine and may extend to one half of the imprisonment for life.

Abetment treated with same gravity as commission of that offence (Section 16), trafficking of children for sexual purposes covered under abetment (Section 16 Explanation III), attempt to commit an offence penalized, for up to half the punishment prescribed for that office (Section 18).

MANDATORY REPORTING

It is mandatory for all persons to report cases of sexual offences against children under Section 19(1), POCSO Act to the local police or the Special Juvenile Police Unit ("SJPU").

It is not mandatory on all persons to report an offence of rape or sexual violence if the survivor is an adult woman. However, hospitals are obliged to inform the police of such incidents under Section 357 C, CrPC.

When and How do I Report an Offence?

You can report an offence by registering a First Information report or on your letterhead with due acknowledgment.

Who and Where to Report?

Section 19 "Reporting of offences", any person (including the child), who has apprehension that an offence under this act, is likely to be committed or has knowledge that such an offence has been committed, shall provide such information to:

- The SJPU; or
- The local police.

How do I File a Private Complaint?

Where?

A Court of Sessions, or the Special Court under the POCSO Act, can take cognizance of a complaint.

Who can File?

Private complaint can be filed by a public servant or by a friend or relative in which response of the local police is to be stated or the fact that the police has not been approached.

FAILURE TO REPORT CASES

Failure to report commission of offence punishable with imprisonment of 6 months or with fine or both [Section 21(1)].

Failure to record an offence is also punishable with imprisonment of 6 months or with fine or both [Section 21(1)].

Failure to report by a person, who is in charge of any company or an institution, in respect of offence committed by subordinate under his control, is also punishable with imprisonment of 1 year and fine [Section 21(2)].

FALSE COMPLAINT

False complaint against any person with malicious intent punishable with imprisonment of 6 months or with fine or both [Section 22(1)]. False complaint against child punishable with imprisonment of 1 year or with fine or with both [Section 22(3)].

No civil or criminal liability for giving information in good faith [Section 19(7)].

DIRECTIONS TO THE MEDIA

Media not to disclose the identity of the child, except when permitted by the Special Court (Section 23). Identity includes: Name, address, photograph, family details, school, neighbourhood or any other particulars which may lead to the disclosure of the identity of the child.

Punishment in case of contravention is imprisonment for not less than 6 months which may extend to 1 year.

PROCEDURES FOR RECORDING STATEMENT OF CHILD

Child friendly procedures (Section 24): Recording at the residence of child. Recording by officer not below the rank of sub inspector. Police officer not to be in uniform. Child should not come in contact with the accused. Child not to be a detained in police station in night.

Recording of the statement of child in the presence of parents or any other person in whom the child has trust and confidence.

Assistance of translator/interpreter/special educator as the case may be [Section 26(2)]. Wherever possible, recording also by audio-video electronic means.

Recording of statement by Magistrate (Section 25): As per Section 164 of CrPC

MEDICAL EXAMINATION OF THE VICTIM

As per Section 164A of CrPC: In case of girl child, medical examination by lady doctor and medical examination should be done in the presence of parents.

In case parent of the child cannot be present, medical examination to be conducted in the presence of a woman nominated by the head of the medical institution. The statement should be recorded as spoken by the child.

ROLE OF MEDICAL EXPERT UNDER SECTION 27

Police shall, as soon as possible, but not later than 24 hours of receiving such information, arrange to take such child to the nearest hospital or medical care facility center for emergency medical care.

Emergency medical care shall be rendered in such a manner as to protect the privacy of the child, and in the presence of the parent or guardian or any other person in whom the child has trust and confidence.

No medical practitioner, hospital or other medical facility center rendering emergency medical care to a child shall demand any legal or magisterial or other documentation as a prerequisite to rendering such care.

EMERGENCY MEDICAL CARE

This includes treatments for cuts, bruises, and other injuries including genital injuries, if any, treatment for exposure to sexually transmitted diseases (STDs) including prophylaxis for identified STDs, treatment for exposure to human immunodeficiency virus (HIV), including prophylaxis for HIV after necessary consultation with infectious disease expert, possible pregnancy and emergency contraceptives should be discussed with the pubertal child and her parent or any other person in whom the child has trust and confidence; and wherever necessary, a referral or consultation for mental or psychological health or other counselling should be made.

Any forensic evidence collected in the course of rendering emergency medical care must be collected in accordance with the Section 27 of the Act. Thus, doctors and support medical staff are involved both at the time of rendering emergency medical care as well as at the time of medical examination.

CONTROVERSIES PUT TO REST

- Confidentiality under the Medical Termination of Pregnancy (MTP) Act 1971

  With mandatory reporting laws in force for rape/sexual assault any such person seeking MTP cannot expect confidentiality of their information because the doctor has to mandatorily inform police before offering MTP services.

- Who shall examine the victim?

  Under Section 164 A CrPC any registered medical Practitioner can examine the person with the consent of that person: Section 27 POCSO insists for a lady doctor to examine when the victim is a girl that is less than 18 years.

- Mandatory reporting when you only suspect child sexual abuse and not confirmed?

  Under Section 19, POCSO reporting is mandatory but many times, the doctor only suspects child sexual abuse and has not confirmed it.

  But Section 19 includes both—offence likely to be committed or committed as to be mandatorily reported.

CONCLUSION

The POCSO Act is gender neutral and provides remedy for all children under 18 years of age, male or female. Abetment or attempt is treated with same gravity as commission of that offence.

Mandatory reporting includes reporting of cases of child sexual abuse even if there is an apprehension that the crime was committed and there is punishment for not reporting.

No medical practitioner, hospital or other medical facility center rendering emergency medical care to a child shall demand any legal or magisterial or other documentation as a prerequisite to rendering such care.

REFERENCES

1. Ministry of Women and Child Development. Model Guidelines under Section 39 of the Protection of Children from Sexual Offences Act, 2012.
2. The Protection of Children from Sexual Offences Act, 2012- Bare act.

CHAPTER 15
Premarital Sex and Unprotected Sexual Activity in Adolescents

Sneha Bhuyar

INTRODUCTION

Premarital sex is having sex, i.e., penetrative vaginal intercourse between couples before formal marriage.

Traditional way of having sex, i.e., only after formal marriage is becoming rare.

The hazards of premarital sex are twofold—unwanted pregnancy and sexually transmitted infections (STIs).

The World Health Organization (WHO) defines adolescence as age group between 10 and 15 years.

It is a period of transformation between childhood to maturity and is characterized by physical, mental, emotional, social, and psychosexual development.

It is a period of rapid growth, exploration, and risk tasking.

In the last decade, boys and even girls have started talking on sex freely, particularly in urban areas. But now it is rapidly spreading toward countryside as well, so many young girls are indulging into sexual activities.

We gynecologists are privileged to counsel the young girls regarding genital hygiene, menstrual hygiene, breast examination, safe sex, and contraception.

Adolescents become anxious about their body image, height, weight, breast size, acne, color, gender discrimination, violence, and many more things which disturb their emotions. They need support, clarification, and encouragement from someone whom they can trust and if they are lacking this, they may be diverted or misguided.

The age of menarche has definitely decreased from 13 to 11 years. These girls reach puberty and physical maturation much sooner in contrast to their emotional maturity. They can be the victims of child abuse, child trafficking which lead to long-term physical and psychological damage.

Adolescence is divided into two parts:
1. *Early adolescence*:
   - Between 10 and 14 years
   - Understanding pubertal changes, awareness of abnormality, anxiety, sociopathology, abnormal growth, and development.
2. *Late adolescence*:
   - Between 15 and 19 years
   - Responsible relationship, responsible sexual behavior, avoiding STIs, and delaying pregnancy
   - Readiness for marriage, readiness for parenthood comes still later.

REASONS FOR PREMARITAL SEX BY TEENAGERS

- Sexual attraction
- Social and media pressure
- Peer pressure
- Desire to be seen by others as normal
- Parental example of permissiveness
- Boredom
- Substance abuse.

As we have already stated that sex before formal marriage is considered as sin in many culture, but nowadays it is widely accepted.

Sex is the normal healthy part of life. It should be fun and pleasurable for both the partners.

As sexual activity releases stress, helps you sleep well, and protects heart, so sexual activity is good for health but it should be safe sex otherwise it can harm both the partners.

What is safe and unsafe sex?

Safe sex: Consensual sexual intercourse with a partner who is not infected with any STIs and involves proper use of contraceptives to prevent pregnancy unless the couple is attempting to have the child.

Unsafe sex/unprotected sex: Sex between the susceptible person and partner who has STIs, without taking measures for its prevention.

Adolescents are impulsive and they have high-risk behavior, more chances of experimenting, having multiple sexual partners, and so more prone for infections like human immunodeficiency virus (HIV) which is the major concern as it is the fourth major cause of mortality in the world.

Premarital sex (unprotected sex) can have many problems:
- Unwanted pregnancy
- Sexually transmitted infections
- As all possibilities are explored before marriage, one tends to lose interest in the partner
- Among partners who have decided to get married, chances of breakup are high
- Even today premarital relationship is not acceptable in society, so you may spoil your image in the society
- *May disturb your mental status*: Worries about unwanted pregnancy, STIs, worries regarding hiding the relationship, and sometimes you regret involving physically sometimes when you are not sure whether the partner is right for you
- Physical and emotional changes may occur when you lose virginity
- When a person gets engaged into premarital sex with one partner and gets married with another partner then the feeling of betrayal, disappointment, and hurt gives emotional burden on you
- One tends to take partner for granted
- It can cause infidelity. Your sexual lust may become unbearable, you might become sex addict, and may not be happy with partner, so risk of multiple partners
- It can change your outlook on love, your partner may break your heart, and may change your attitude toward love. You may view all relations with suspicion.

Apart from premarital sex, people can have fornication where two peoples not married to each other can have consensual sex. When one of the two partners is married to someone else, it is described as adultery.

What is unprotected sex/unsafe sex?
- Multiple partners
- Anal sex
- Sex and drugs
- Paying for sex
- Unprotected sex—vaginal, oral, and anal sex without condoms
- If condoms are used, risk of transmission of HIV and STIs
- Definitely people who have sex with multiple sexual partners have higher risk of transmission of STIs.

ANAL SEX

Anal sex is most risky because of the anatomical reason as anal lining is very thin.

How to protect?
Using condoms with lubrication can reduce but cannot prevent.

DRUGS

Not only sexual activity but intravenous (IV) drug abuse as well can lead to transmission of HIV, hepatitis, etc.

How to protect?
Avoid having sex with IV drug abusers.

PAYING FOR SEX

Because the partners who are doing it for money, food, and shelter, they have multiple partners and so it is high-risk sex.

What measures can be taken for minimizing these problems?
Measures taken for minimizing these problems are described in **Flowchart 1**.

What measures can be taken after having unprotected intercourse?
- Weeing immediately after sexual intercourse and washing thoroughly can minimize risk of urinary tract infection (within first 30 minutes).
- Wash the area around genitalia gently with plain warm water or mild soap, but if you have sensitive skin or infection, it may irritate or worsen the situation.
- *Within first 72 hours*: Take emergency contraceptive pills. The emergency contraceptive pill can be taken up to 72 hours, i.e., 3 days after unprotected intercourse. Recent research has shown that it can be effective within 4 days of unprotected intercourse.
- If it is late than 3 days, then intrauterine contraceptive device can be inserted.
- For STIs, you need to get investigated after 2 weeks.
- After 3 weeks, do a pregnancy test or serum β-human chorionic gonadotropin (β-hCG) levels.
- For next time, always organize your contraceptive beforehand.
- For prevention of pregnancy, oral contraceptives or intrauterine devices (IUDs) are better, but for STIs barrier methods—condoms are the best, so it should be in addition.

SEXUALITY EDUCATION

- Would sexuality education help?
- Should girls and boys be educated together?
- What are the advantages?
- What is the proper timing for giving sexuality education?
- Having proper knowledge and understanding about the process will reduce curiosity and experimenting.

Aims of Sexuality Education
- To have proper understanding of physical and psychological changes

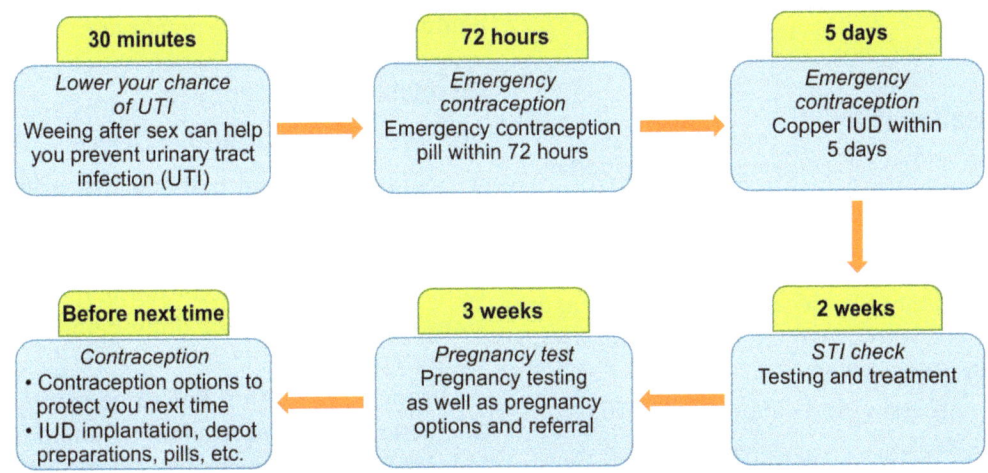

Flowchart 1: Measures taken for minimizing unprotected sex.

(IUD: intrauterine device; STI: sexually transmitted infection)
(*Source:* Bhalerao-Gandhi A, Biniwale P. Gynecological Manual on Adolescent Girls and Young Women, 1st edition. New Delhi: Jaypee Brothers Medical Publishers (P) Ltd.; 2009).

- Positive attitude toward sexuality and relationship
- To avoid STIs and acquired immunodeficiency syndrome (AIDS)
- Awareness about sexual abuse
- Avoidance of unwanted pregnancy
- It should be an ongoing process starting at age 10 years from home before they become curious and gather information.

Who can give sexuality education?
Doctors, nurses, psychologists, and social workers can give sexuality education.

Points to Remember during Sexuality Education
- Avoid unscientific answers
- Emotional involvement
- Judgmental attitude
- Too much intimacy
- Body contact
- Naked pictures
- Late hours of training
- Religious or cultural criticism
- Vulgar jokes.

What all it should include?
- Growth and development
- Sexual behavior
- Personal skills
- Relationships
- Sexual health
- Society and culture.

- *Growth and development*:
  - Basic structure and function of reproductive system
  - Changes during adolescence
  - Body image, gender identity
  - Reproduction
  - Pregnancy and delivery.
- *Sexuality*:
  - Adolescent sexuality
  - Abstinence
  - Masturbation
  - Homosexuality
  - Differences in sexuality.

How is the ability to cope up with situation?
- Values
- Decision-making
- Communication
- Negotiation
- Seeking help during distress.
- *Relationships*:
  - With family
  - With friends
  - Girl-boy relationship.
- *Sexual health*:
  - Nutrition
  - Physical health
  - Reproductive health and hygiene
  - Adolescent problems
  - Sexual and substance abuse
  - Sexually transmitted infections, HIV/AIDS.

- *Society and culture*:
  - Sexuality of society
  - Myths about sexuality
  - Laws about sexuality.

Sexuality Education in India

Cultural, religious, and social factors are of prime importance in India. Sexuality education is not acceptable widely in India and that is the reason, it cannot be made compulsory or as part of the curriculum. Secondly, some people are so staunch that they cannot even accept the name as sexuality education, so it needs to be named as *adolescent health education/family life education*.

Gender, age, necessity, and culture—all these factors need to be considered.

This kind of education should start from 10 years of age, so we need to divide the adolescents into two groups:
- First group: 10–14 years
- Second group: 15–19 years.

It should be graded education, whatever is needed for their age group should be provided.

Definitely permission from parents, teachers, and school authorities is required.

Questionnaire should be provided to them for filling personally without mentioning names. Pretesting, pilot studies, and feedback are essential.

Repetitions and reinforcements should be there.

Child marriages, female feticide, gender bias, one-sided love, population explosion, and sexual abuse—all these issues should be addressed.

The main aim of sexuality education should be behavioral and social change.

As girls are shy and feel embarrassed easily, separate sessions should be arranged so that they can understand the subject thoroughly and can ask their queries.

Sexuality education and advice regarding appropriate contraception are the two effective measures for reducing the problems related to premarital sex.

■ CHOICE OF CONTRACEPTIVES

Natural Methods

Knowledge about fertile period and safe period, regularity of cycle, simultaneously washing effectively after intercourse, and using spermicidal jellies should be better.

Barrier Methods

Male and female condoms.

Oral Contraceptives

Regular/emergency, preferably the newer low-dose contraceptives should be preferred.

Injectable Contraceptives

Intrauterine Contraceptive Device

It should be successful, cost-effective, easily available, and should not have side effects.

Detailed personal, family, and medical history is to be taken and detailed examination along with Pap smear should preferably done before starting the oral contraceptives.

Proper preparation has to be selected and proper instructions regarding regular consumption of the pills are to be given, otherwise chances of side effects will be high.

The *newer oral contraceptives* which should be used for adolescents are:
- Second-generation norgestrel
- Ethynodiol diacetate
- Norethindrone
- Levonorgestrel
- Third-generation norgestimate
- Desogestrel
- Spironolactone derivatives
- Drospirenone
- Antiandrogens
- Cyproterone acetate.

■ WORLD HEALTH ORGANIZATION ADOLESCENT HEALTH AND DEVELOPMENT INITIATIVES

Adolescent age group is generally considered healthy as mortality in this age group is low, but mortality statistics alone cannot describe health status.

Adolescents are still growing and developing and they need holistic support as physical, psychosocial, sexual, and reproductive development makes them vulnerable to the health hazards.

Adolescents are having lack of knowledge about their needs and illnesses.

Unaware of consequences.

May not want to seek attention or help.

May not know where to go and seek advice, help, counseling, and treatment.

If there are no opportunities for all these things, then there is definitely missed opportunities for prevention of health problems through early detection and prompt treatment.

Facts to be Accepted about Indian Adolescents

- More than 45% girls are married by 18 years of age
- Girls are the ones to have sex at an earlier age as they get married earlier
- Contraception use rate is 22.5% in adolescents
- Earlier age of pregnancy
- 16% have started childbearing by 16–19 years
- Maternal mortality is two to five times higher
- Infant mortality is twice the general population (77/1,000 live births)
- *Malnutrition*: Undernutrition in two-thirds of adolescents and 10% overnutrition in adolescents
- About 35% of new HIV infections in adolescents.

At present, the adolescent health services are not adolescent friendly and they do not meet the needs and expectations of adolescents.

Private practitioners like gynecologist and pediatrician should be able to extend their services as adolescent friendly health services (AFHS).

Medical, social, psychological, and behavioral dimensions should be added to AFHS.

Perception of body image, peer pressure, smoking, drinking, sexuality, and attraction about opposite sex.

How should adolescent friendly health services be modeled?

- Should be affordable and acceptable as per the local customs
- Should be available for all adolescent irrespective of gender and marital status
- There should be comprehensive package as per felt need of adolescents and should be tailor-made
- Linkages with other institution to promote publicity and encourage utilization
- There should be strict policies on privacy and confidentiality
- Training of peer counselor so as to convey key message.

How should be the clinic?

- Environment should be pleasant
- Registration should not be compulsory
- Timings should be separate as far as privacy is concerned
- Provider's attitude should be nonjudgmental
- Information, education, and counseling material should be adequately available.

What all services should be available?

- Administrative
- Antenatal
- Nutrition
- Gynecological care
- Family welfare
- Preventive
- Education
- Laboratory services.

CONCLUSION

Having sex is a natural instinct, there is nothing wrong. Sex releases stress, helps the heart as well provided it is protected and safe sex.

If it is unsafe sex, i.e., anal sex, oral sex, sex with multiple partners, sex with high-risk partners, or paid sex, then it is definitely hazardous for health.

Premarital sex has multiple fold risks but most important are:

- Unwanted pregnancy
- Sexually transmitted infections.

To avoid these problems, adolescents should be provided with proper information, counseling, and that is the reason, there is a felt need of *adolescent friendly health clinics or centers*.

SUGGESTED READING

1. Bhalerao-Gandhi A, Biniwale P. Gynecological Manual on Adolescent Girls and Young Women, 1st edition. New Delhi: Jaypee Brothers Medical Publishers (P) Ltd.; 2009.
2. Centers for Disease Control and Prevention (CDC) (2002). Sexually Transmitted Diseases Treatment Guidelines. [online] Available from: https://www.cdc.gov/mmwr/preview/mmwrhtml/rr5106a1.htm. [Last accessed April, 2020].
3. Dennis KJ, Elstein M. Education in sexuality in the medical curriculum. Clin Obstet Gynaecol. 1980;7:183-91.
4. Dickson KE, Ashton J, Smith J. Does setting adolescent-friendly standards improve the quality of care in clinics? Evidence from South Africa. Int J Qual Health Care. 2007;19:80-9.
5. Kothari P. Common Sexual Problems...Solutions, 2nd edition. New Delhi: UBS Publishers Distributors; 1994.
6. Panthaki D. Education in Human Sexuality: A Sourcebook for Educators. Mumbai: Family Planning Association of India; 1998.
7. World Health Organization (WHO) (2002). Adolescent Friendly Health Services: An Agenda for Change. [online] Available from: https://apps.who.int/iris/bitstream/handle/10665/67923/WHO_FCH_CAH_02.14.pdf?sequence=1&isAllowed=y. [Last accessed April, 2020].

CHAPTER 16

Adolescent-friendly Health Clinics

Vaishali Chavan, Varsha Lahade

INTRODUCTION

- More than 1.1 million adolescents aged 10–19 years died in 2016, over 3,000 every day, mostly from preventable or treatable causes.
- Road traffic injuries were the leading cause of death among adolescents in 2016. Other major causes of adolescent deaths include suicide, interpersonal violence, human immunodeficiency virus/acquired immunodeficiency syndrome (HIV/AIDS), and diarrheal diseases.
- Half of all mental health disorders in adulthood start by age 14 years, but most cases are undetected and untreated.
- Globally, there are 44 births per 1,000 to girls aged 15–19 years per year.

Around 1.2 billion people or one in six of the world's population are adolescents aged 10–19 years. Most are healthy, but there is still substantial premature death, illness, and injury among adolescents. Illnesses can hinder their ability to grow and develop to their full potential. Alcohol or tobacco use, lack of physical activity, unprotected sex, and/or exposure to violence can jeopardize not only their current health, but also their health as adults and even the health of their future children.

Promoting healthy behaviors during adolescence and taking steps to better protect young people from health risks are critical for the prevention of health problems in adulthood and for countries' future health and ability to develop and thrive.

MAIN HEALTH ISSUES

Injuries

Unintentional injuries are the leading cause of death and disability among adolescents. In 2016, over 135,000 adolescents died as a result of road traffic accidents. Young drivers need advice on driving safely while laws that prohibit driving under the influence of alcohol and drugs need to be strictly enforced.

Mental Health

Depression is one of the leading causes of illness and disability among adolescents and suicide is the second leading cause of death in adolescents. Violence, poverty, humiliation, and feeling devalued can increase the risk of developing mental health problems.

Programs to help strengthen the ties between adolescents and their families are also important.

Violence

Interpersonal violence is the third leading cause of death in adolescents. Promoting nurturing relationships between parents and children early in life, providing training in life skills, and reducing access to alcohol and firearms can help to prevent injuries and deaths due to violence.

Human Immunodeficiency Virus/Acquired Immunodeficiency Syndrome

An estimated 2.1 million adolescents were living with HIV in 2016, the great majority in the World Health Organization (WHO) African region. One of the specific targets of the health Sustainable Development Goal-3 (SDG-3)[1] is that by 2030, there should be an end to the epidemics of AIDS, tuberculosis, malaria and neglected tropical diseases, hepatitis, waterborne diseases, and other communicable diseases

Diarrhea and lower respiratory tract infections are estimated to be among the top 10 causes of death for 10–19-year-old.

Early Pregnancy and Childbirth

The leading cause of death for 15–19-year-old girls globally is complications from pregnancy and childbirth. One of the specific targets of the health SDG-3 is that by 2030, the world should ensure universal access to sexual and reproductive healthcare services including for family planning, information and education, and the integration of reproductive health into national strategies and programs. Better access to contraceptive information and services can reduce the number of girls becoming pregnant and giving birth at too young an age. Laws that are enforced that specify a minimum age of marriage at 18 years can help.

Alcohol and Drugs

Harmful drinking among adolescents is a major concern. Drug use among 15–19-year-old is also an important global concern. Drug control may focus on reducing drug demand, drug supply, or both and successful programs usually include structural, community, and individual-level interventions.

Nutrition and Micronutrient Deficiencies

Iron deficiency anemia was the second leading cause of years lost by adolescents to death and disability in 2016. Iron and folic acid supplements are a solution that also helps to promote health before adolescents become parents.

Undernutrition and Obesity

Many boys and girls in developing countries enter adolescence undernourished, making them more vulnerable to disease and early death.

Physical Activity

Physical activity provides fundamental health benefits for adolescents including improved cardiorespiratory and muscular fitness, bone health, maintenance of a healthy body weight, and psychosocial benefits. The WHO recommends for adolescents to accumulate at least 60 minutes of moderate-to-vigorous intensity physical activity daily, which may include play, games, and sports, but also activity for transportation (such as cycling and walking) or physical education.

■ RIGHTS OF ADOLESCENTS

The rights of children (people under 18 years of age) to survive, grow, and develop are enshrined in international legal documents. In 2013, the Committee on the Rights of the Child (CRC), which oversees the child rights convention, published guidelines on the right of children and adolescents to the enjoyment of the highest attainable standard of health and a general comment on realizing the rights of children during adolescence was published in 2016. It highlights states' obligations to recognize the special health and development needs and rights of adolescents and young people.

■ REFERENCE

1. United Nations Statistics Division. (2019). Sustainable Development Goals Indicators. [online] Available from: https://unstats.un.org/sdgs/indicators/database/?indicator=3.7.2. [Last accessed April, 2020]

Index

Page numbers followed by *f* refer to figure, *fc* refer to flowchart, and *t* refer to table.

A

Abdominal pain, symptoms of 12
Abdomino-pelvic pain, chronic 17
Abnormal uterine 36
    bleeding 4, 37, 40, 61
Abortion 42, 43
    unsafe 2, 44, 64
Absolute uterine factors 1
Abstinence 61
Acne 36
Acquired anatomical abnormalities 1
Acquired immunodeficiency syndrome 54, 71, 74
Acute bleeding, management of 37
Acyclovir 57
Adenomas 12
Adolescent friendly health services 73
Adolescent health 65
    programs 46
Adolescent pregnancy 44, 49
Adolescent reproductive program 2
Adolescent responsive quality healthcare 2
Adolescent-friendly health clinics 74
Adult endometriosis 32, 33
    phenotype of 33*t*
Affect future fertility 39
Age-related fecundity decline 1
Alcohol and drugs 75
Alkylating agents 23
Alpha-fetoprotein 24
Alpha-hydroxylase deficiency 1, 12
Alpha-reductase deficiency 12
Amenorrhea 11
    causes of primary 11, 13*t*, 14*t*
    evaluation of primary 12, 14*fc*
    primary 11, 12, 13, 15
Ampicillin 58
Anal sex 70
Androgen insensitivity syndrome 1, 12, 15
Androstenedione 3
Anemia 15, 48
    causes of 48
    global burden 48
    management of 51, 51*t*
    mild 51
    moderate 51
    presentation of 49
    prevention of 49, 50*fc*
    severe 51
    signs and symptoms of 49
    treatment of 50
Anogenital warts 2
Anomalies affecting uterus 16
Anorchia 1
Anorectal malformations 1
Anorexia nervosa 12, 15
Antepartum hemorrhage 60
Antiandrogens 72
Antifibrinolytics 39
Anti-müllerian hormone 3
Anxiety 2
Arcuate uterus 16, 16*f*
Aromatase deficiency 1, 12
Artificial ovary 26
Asherman's syndrome 1
Autoimmune ovarian insufficiency 2
Azithromycin 57

B

Bacterial vaginosis 54, 57
Balanced diet 49
Barrier contraception 61
Benzathine penicillin G 58
Bichloroacetic acid 57
Bicornuate uterus 16, 17*f*
Bilateral cryptorchidism 1
Blood pressure 3
Body mass index 3
Bone age, tests for 3
Borderline ovarian tumors 24
Boredom 69
BRCA mutation 25
Breast
    absent 13
    development 3
    present 13
Breastfeeding difficulties 45
Bruising, history of 37

C

Calymmatobacterium granulomatis 55
Cancer
    adolescents with 5
    diagnosis 22
Carcinosarcomas 25
Cardiac disease, end-stage 2
Cefotetan 58
Ceftriaxone 57, 58
Central nervous system 13
Cerebral palsy 1
Cervical
    atresia 1
    inflammation 55
Cervicitis 57
Chancroid 54, 55
Chemotherapy 23
Child friendly procedures 67
Children from Sexual Offences Act, protection of 60, 66
Chlamydia 2, 37, 54
    infection 54, 57
    trachomatis 54
Clindamycin 57
Combined oral contraceptive pill 33, 38, 61
Community education 45
Complete blood count 51
Congenital adrenal hyperplasia 1
    adult-onset 12
Congenital anomalies 16
Congenital central nervous system defects 1
Congenital lipoid adrenal hyperplasia 12
Congestive cardiac failure 49
Contraception 45, 60, 62
    injectable 62, 72
Contraceptives
    choice of 72
    long-acting reversible 61
Craniopharyngioma 2, 12
Cryotherapy 57
Cushing's disease 12
Cushing's syndrome 2
Cyclic hormone thermotherapy 35
Cyproterone acetate 72
Cystic fibrosis 1
Cytomegalovirus 54

D

Danazol 33
Dating violence 2
Davydov procedure 21
Deep vein thrombosis 38
Dehydroepiandrosterone sulfate 3, 13, 38
Delivery and postpartum 45
Deoxyribonucleic acid 23
Depression 2, 74
Desogestrel 72
Diabetes
    mellitus 2
    screening for 3
Diarrheal diseases 74
Down's syndrome 1
Doxycycline 57, 58
Drospirenone 72

E

Eating disorders 2
Embryo cryopreservation 22

Emergency contraception 61, 62
Emergency medical care 68
Empty sella 2
    turcica 12
Endocrine disrupting chemicals 2
Endocrinological disorders 15
Endometriosis 1, 5, 31*f*
    classification of 34*f*
    pathophysiology of 32*f*
Enzyme deficiencies 12, 15
Epididymitis 57
Epithelial ovarian cancer 23
Epithelial tumors 25
Erythrocyte sedimentation rate 3
Erythromycin 57
    ethylsuccinate 57
Ethinyl estradiol 38
Ethynodiol diacetate 72
Eugonadotropic eugonadism 12, 15
European Society for Medical Oncology 25
European Society of Human Reproduction and Embryology 26

F

False complaint 67
Famciclovir 57
Female intersex 12
Feminine sprays 2
Fertility awareness method 62
Fertility preservation 26*fc*
    facilities 2
Fertility-sparing
    methods 22
    strategies 25*fc*
    surgery 23, 25
Fertiprotective agents 23, 26
Fetal growth restriction 17
Fibroids 1, 28
Folic acid supplementation 50
Follicle-stimulating hormone 1, 11, 12, 14
Forbes-Albright syndrome 12
Fragile-X permutation 1
Frasier syndrome 14

G

Galactosemia 1, 12
Genetic disorders 12
Genital herpes 55
    simplex 57
Genital mutilation 1
Genital tract examination 3
Genital trauma and mutilation 2
Genital tuberculosis 2
Genital warts 55, 57
Germ cell
    damage 26
    tumors 2, 22, 23
Gonadal dysgenesis 1, 11, 13, 14
Gonadoblastoma 14

Gonadotoxic chemotherapy 2
Gonadotropin levels, classification on 11
Gonadotropin-releasing hormone 13, 14, 23, 26, 35
    agonists 33
    deficiency 1, 12
    receptor mutation 12
Gonadotropin-resistant ovary syndrome 12
Gonococcal infections 57
Gonorrhea 53, 54
    prevalence of 54
Granuloma inguinale 54, 55
Gynecological cancers 22

H

Haemophilus ducreyi 55
Health concern 43
Hematocolpos 20
Hematometra 20
Hematosalpinx 20
Hemivagina 17
Hemoglobin 38, 48
Hemogram 3
Hepatitis 54
Herpes simplex 54
Hirsutism 36
    signs of 3
Hookworm
    prevention of 50
    treatment of 50
Hormonal medical therapy 39
Human chorionic gonadotropin 38
Human immunodeficiency virus 43, 54, 60, 68, 69, 74
Human papillomavirus 53, 58
    infection 2, 54, 55
Human rights, universal declaration of 64
Hymen, anomalies of 18
Hyperandrogenemia 4
Hypergonadotropic hypogonadism 11, 13
Hypergonadotropic states 14
Hyperprolactinemia 2, 15
Hyperthyroidism 2
Hypogonadotropic hypogonadism 2, 15
Hypogonadotropic states 14
Hypopituitarism 1
Hypothalamic dysfunction 36
Hypothalamic hypogonadism 12
Hypothyroidism 2
Hysterectomized women 26
Hysteroscopic metroplasty 16

I

Imiquimod 57
Imperforate hymen 1, 12, 15, 18, 19*f*
In vitro ovarian follicle
    growth 26
    maturation 26
Infection 2, 43

Infertility 43
Inguinal canal, examination of 3
Insulin-like growth factor-1 13
International Conference on Population and Development Programme of Action 64
International Federation of Gynecology and Obstetrics 23
Interpersonal violence 74
Intrauterine
    balloon 39
    contraceptive device 62, 72
    device 70, 71
    system 62
Ipsilateral renal agenesis 17
Iron
    deficiency anemia 48, 50
    requirement, increased 48
    supplementation 49
Ivermectin 57, 58

J

Juvenile Justice Act 66
Juvenile police unit 60

K

Kallmann's syndrome 1, 12, 15
Kidney function test 3
Klinefelter's syndrome 1

L

Leiomyomas, etiology of 28
Leptin deficiency 2
Levofloxacin 57
Levonorgestrel 72
    intrauterine system 62
Lichen planus 2
Lichen sclerosis 2
Liver
    disease, end-stage 2
    function test 3
Local irritants, use of 2
Lung disease, end-stage 2
Luteinizing hormone 1, 13, 14, 23
Lymphadenopathy 3
Lymphoblastic leukemia, acute 2
Lymphogranuloma venereum 54, 55, 57

M

Maintenance therapy 40
Malaria 2
    parasite testing 51
Malnutrition 12, 15, 73
Mayer-Rokitansky-Küster-Hauser syndrome 1, 12, 15, 20, 20*f*
Mcindoe
    procedure 15
    vaginoplasty 20

Medical Termination of Pregnancy Act 68
Medroxyprogesterone acetate 13, 62
Menses, normal and abnormal 36
Menstrual abnormalities 36, 40
Menstrual bleeding 36
    pathophysiology of 11
Menstrual hygiene 2, 65
Mental and psychological state 2
Mental health 74
    disorders 74
Metabolic and endocrinological problems 1
Metronidazole 57, 58
Mixed connective tissue disease 2
Mosaicism 14
Mosaics 11
Mucopurulent cervicitis 55
Müllerian agenesis 13, 15, 20
    diagnosis of 4
Müllerian anomalies 1, 4, 15
Müllerian development
    absence of 12
    normal 12
Müllerian ducts 19
Mullerian dysgenesis 1
Müllerian tumors 25
Multiple partners 70
Mumps 2
Myeloid leukemia, acute 2
Myxedema 49

N

National Commission for Protection of Children's Rights 66
Neisseria gonorrhoeae 4, 55
Neoplasia 2
Neuroblastoma 2
Nondysgerminomatous tumors 24
Nongonococcal urethritis 55, 57
Non-Hodgkin lymphoma 2
Nonobstructed cervix 17
Nonpharmacological management 39
Nonsteroidal anti-inflammatory drugs 33, 35, 38
Norethindrone 72
Norgestimate, third-generation 72
Norgestrel, second-generation 72
Nutrition and micronutrient deficiencies 75

O

Obesity 1, 36, 75
Obstetric complications 43
Ofloxacin 57
Oocyte
    cryopreservation 22
    immature 22
Oophoropexy 23
Oral contraceptive 39, 70, 72
Ovarian cancer 22, 25
Ovarian cryopreservation 22

Ovarian cysts 5
Ovarian deficiency, primary 1
Ovarian failure
    premature 2
    prevention of chemotherapy-associated 23
Ovarian germ cell tumors, malignant 23
Ovarian hyperstimulation, controlled 22
Ovarian reserve, predicting 23
Ovarian teratoma, immature 24
Ovarian transposition 23
Ovarian tumors 2, 22, 23
Ovulatory dysfunction 36

P

Pediculosis pubis 57
Peer pressure 69
Pelvic examination 13
Pelvic inflammatory disease 54, 55, 58, 60
    chronic 2
Pelvic irradiation 2
Pelvic pain, chronic 43
Perineal wash 2
Periodic abstinence method 62
Peripheral blood smear, examination of 51
Permethrin 57, 58
Physical activity 75
Pineal gland tumors 12
Piperonyl butoxide 57
Pituitary adenoma 2
Pituitary hypoplasia 12
Platelet count 3
Podofilox 57
Polycystic ovary syndrome 1, 4, 12, 38, 61
Poor perineal hygiene 2
Poor socioeconomic status 2
Postabortal sepsis 2
Prader orchidometer 3
Prader-Willi's syndrome 2
Pregnancy
    hypertensive disorders of 60
    prevention of 70
    unwanted 64, 69, 70
Premarital sex 69
Premature deliveries 60
Progestins 33
Prolactinomas 12
Prostaglandin synthesis inhibitors 39
Pseudohypoparathyroidism 2
Psychological stress 2
Puberty 53
    completion of 36
Pulmonary embolism 38
Pure dysgerminoma 24
Pure gonadal dysgenesis 11, 14
Pyrethrins 57

R

Radical surgery 25
Radiotherapy 23

Receptor and enzyme defects 1
Renal disease 49
    end-stage 2
Reproductive age, women of 26*fc*
Reproductive tract anomalies 4
Respiratory illness 49
Rheumatoid arthritis 2

S

Salpingectomy 25
Savage syndrome 12
Scabies 54, 58
Septate uterus 16, 16*f*
Serum
    alpha-fetoprotein 24
    anti-müllerian hormone 23
    estradiol 3
    thyroid-stimulating hormone 13
Sex
    and drugs 70
    chromosomes
        abnormal 11, 13
        normal 11
    cord stromal tumors, malignant 24
    paying for 70
    safe 69
    unprotected 69, 70
    unsafe 69, 70
Sexual abuse 44
Sexual activity, unprotected 69
Sexual and reproductive health 64
Sexual attraction 69
Sexual characters, development of 12
Sexual health 71
    program 2
    thieves of 1
Sexual history 37
Sexuality 2
    education 70–72
Sexually transmitted
    diseases 4, 53, 60, 68
    infection 2, 44, 53, 55, 56, 60, 64, 69–71
Sheehan's syndrome 2
Sigmoid vaginoplasty 21
Simmonds disease 12
Social and media pressure 69
Soft tissue 2
Soil transmitted helminths 50
Sphingosine-1-phosphate 26
Spina bifida 1
Spinal injuries 1
Spironolactone derivatives 72
Spontaneous abortion 17
    risk for 16
State Commission for Protection of Children's Right 66
Steroid-dependent nephrotic syndrome 2
Stress 12
Subseptate uterus 16
Substance abuse 69
Suicide 74

Sulbactam 58
Swyer's syndrome 1, 11, 14
Syphilis 54, 55, 58
    prevalence of 55

T

Teenage pregnancies 42, 60
    management of 45
Testicular regression 1
Testicular tumors 2
Tetanus 43
Thyroid
    disease 12
    function tests 3
    stimulating hormone 13, 14
Thyromegaly 3
Tinidazole 57, 58
Tranexamic acid 39
Transgender 2
Transverse vaginal septum 1, 12, 15, 19
    types of 19*f*
Treponema pallidum 55
Trichloroacetic acid 57
Trichomonas vaginalis 55
Trichomoniasis 54, 58
True intersex 12
Tumor 2
    marker 3
Turner's syndrome 1, 11, 13

U

Undernutrition 75
Unhygienic conditions 43
Unicornuate uterus 17, 18*f*
Urethral discharge, abnormal 55
Urethral inflammation 55
Urological tract examination 3
Uterine artery embolization 29
Uterine cavity 18*f*
Uterine evacuation 40
Uterine fibroid 28, 29
    pathophysiology 29*f*
Uterine leiomyomas 28
Uterine leiomyomata 28*f*
Uterine rupture 18
Uterus 43
    and vagina, congenital absence of 1
    didelphys 17, 17*f*, 19*f*
    present 13
    transplantation 26

V

Vagina, anomalies of 19
Vaginal agenesis 20
    diagnosis of 21
    differential diagnosis of 20
Vaginoplasty 15
Valacyclovir 57
Vasculitis 2
Vecchietti procedure 21
Violence 74
Virilisation, signs of 3
Vision 3
Visual examination 13
Visual field 3
Vitamin A 43
von Willebrand disease 3
Vulvovaginitis 2

W

Weight loss 12
Williams surgery 15
Williams vulvovaginoplasty 21

X

X chromosome, abnormal 11

Y

Y chromosome 1
Yolk sac tumors 24

EU GSPR Authorised Reprsentative
Logos Europe, 9 rue Nicolas Poussin
1700, La Rochelle, France
Phone: +33 (0) 6 67 93 73 78
E-mail: contact@logoseurope.eu

www.ingramcontent.com/pod-product-compliance
Ingram Content Group UK Ltd.
Pitfield, Milton Keynes, MK11 3LW, UK
UKHW050431150426
5217IPUK00019B/1338